Understanding Fertility

T0028635

Infertility can have devastating physical, emotional and financial effects on people affected. It is a common problem, but can be hard to talk about and hard to understand. In this concise book, Dr Kovacs, a reproductive gynae-cologist who has spent the past 40 years working with patients facing fertility problems, focuses on and unpicks key misconceptions. In his clear explan-ations, he covers the basic physiology of conceiving and describes the areas that have to be explored for those who have not yet been able to conceive. Specific chapters cover the three major problem areas: lack of releasing eggs, sperm problems and abnormalities of the female passages. Treatment options are discussed for each of these areas, including technical details and a brief readable overview of their history. The many ways of parenting, which are now available are also detailed. This is a recommended read for couples wanting to conceive, their friends and families, and anyone who wants to understand fertility.

Gab Kovacs is a reproductive gynaecologist with over 40 years of clinical experience and Professor of Obstetrics and Gynaecology at Monash University, Melbourne, Australia. He was a member of the Monash University IVF team that produced the world's 4th–13th IVF babies. He is Honorary Life Member of the International Federation of Fertility Societies and The Fertility Society of Australia.

The *Understanding Life* series is for anyone wanting an engaging and concise way into a key biological topic. Offering a multidisciplinary perspective, these accessible guides address common misconceptions and misunderstandings in a thoughtful way to help stimulate debate and encourage a more in-depth understanding. Written by leading thinkers in each field, these books are for anyone wanting an expert overview that will enable clearer thinking on each topic.

Series Editor: Kostas Kampourakis http://kampourakis.com

Published titles:

Understanding Evolution	Kostas Kampourakis	9781108746083
Understanding Coronavirus	Raul Rabadan	9781108826716
Understanding Development	Alessandro Minelli	9781108799232
Understanding Evo-Devo	Wallace Arthur	9781108819466
Understanding Genes	Kostas Kampourakis	9781108812825
Understanding DNA Ancestry	Sheldon Krimsky	9781108816038
Understanding Intelligence	Ken Richardson	9781108940368
Understanding Metaphors in the Life Sciences	Andrew S. Reynolds	9781108940498
Understanding Cancer	Robin Hesketh	9781009005999
Understanding How Science Explains the World	Kevin McCain	9781108995504
Understanding Race	Rob DeSalle and Ian Tattersall	9781009055581
Understanding Human Evolution	Ian Tattersall	9781009101998
Understanding Human Metabolism	Keith N. Frayn	9781009108522
Understanding Fertility	Gab Kovacs	9781009054164

Forthcoming:

Understanding Forensic DNA	Suzanne Bell and John M. Butler	9781009044011
Understanding Natural Selection	Michael Ruse	9781009088329
Understanding Creationism	Glenn Branch	9781108927505
Understanding Species	John S. Wilkins	9781108987196
Understanding the Nature–Nurture Debate	Eric Turkheimer	9781108958165

Understanding Fertility

GAB KOVACS
Monash University Medical School

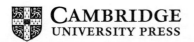

CAMBRIDGE
UNIVERSITY PRESS

University Printing House, Cambridge CB2 8BS, United Kingdom

One Liberty Plaza, 20th Floor, New York, NY 10006, USA

477 Williamstown Road, Port Melbourne, VIC 3207, Australia

314–321, 3rd Floor, Plot 3, Splendor Forum, Jasola District Centre, New Delhi – 110025, India

103 Penang Road, #05–06/07, Visioncrest Commercial, Singapore 238467

Cambridge University Press is part of the University of Cambridge.

It furthers the University's mission by disseminating knowledge in the pursuit of education, learning, and research at the highest international levels of excellence.

www.cambridge.org
Information on this title: www.cambridge.org/9781316511626
DOI: 10.1017/9781009053396

© Cambridge University Press 2022

First published 2022

Printed in the United Kingdom by TJ Books Limited, Padstow Cornwall

A catalogue record for this publication is available from the British Library.

Library of Congress Cataloging-in-Publication Data
Names: Kovacs, Gabor, 1947 April 6– author.
Title: Understanding fertility / Gab Kovacs, Monash University Medical School.
Description: Cambridge, United Kingdom ; New York, NY : Cambridge University Press, 2022. |
    Series: Understanding life | Includes bibliographical references and index.
Identifiers: LCCN 2021062719 (print) | LCCN 2021062720 (ebook) | ISBN 9781316511626 (hardback) |
    ISBN 9781009054164 (paperback) | ISBN 9781009053396 (epub)
Subjects: LCSH: Fertility. | Fertility, Human. | Pregnancy.
Classification: LCC QP251 .K685 2022 (print) | LCC QP251 (ebook) | DDC 612.6/2–dc23/eng/20220111
LC record available at https://lccn.loc.gov/2021062719
LC ebook record available at https://lccn.loc.gov/2021062720

ISBN 978-1-316-51162-6 Hardback
ISBN 978-1-009-05416-4 Paperback

'Dealing with infertility can be stressful and time consuming, often compounded by a lack of understanding due to inadequate explanations. This book interprets all the medical and technical language; it explains the terminology, the problems and their treatments simply and understandably. Unusually, in discussing many specific points, it acknowledges that there is no clear answer, but describes the different views and provides a conclusion. There are no simplistic explanations – rather, this is a book for those who want to know all the details. It is well illustrated and provides a balanced perspective on contemporary approaches to the management of infertility.'

> Professor Ian Cooke, University of Sheffield, UK, and Chairman (1996–9) and later President (2001–4) of the British Fertility Society

'This is a much needed and long-awaited book which uncovers in a clear and comprehensive way the physiology and pathophysiology of human fertility. Written by one of the world's pioneers of reproductive medicine, the book can serve as an invaluable asset for any person facing fertility issues.'

> Professor Ariel Weissman, IVF Unit, Edith Wolfson Medical Center, Holon, and Faculty of Medicine, Tel Aviv University, Tel Aviv, Israel

'Although written for patients, *Understanding Fertility* contains descriptions of issues associated with fertility that are basic and sophisticated.

I personally acquired many new insights. Patients will find the concepts in this book easy to comprehend fully. The illustrations and graphics are beautifully executed.

This is a must-read for anyone undergoing fertility treatment, but anyone interested in reproduction who read this book will find their time was well spent. The author is an iconic expert.'

> Alan Decherney MD, Editor-In-Chief, *Global Reproductive Health*, the journal of the International Federation of Fertility Societies (IFFS)

I would like to dedicate this book to four of my mentors, four of my many outstanding teachers - Henry Burger, Carl Wood, David de Kretser and John Leeton

Contents

Colour plates can be found between pages 78 and 79.

Foreword

Sex and reproduction are more broadly and openly discussed nowadays than ever before. Still, there are numerous misunderstandings about when a woman could become pregnant, and even more about why a woman cannot become pregnant. In the latter case, frustration and disappointment often accompany the failed attempts of couples to have a child, initially by natural means of procreation and then by what is described as assisted reproduction methods. Unfortunately, what seems simple and straightforward for some couples is painful and stressful for others. There exist couples who have tried for years to have a baby, without success. Some people suggest that adoption is an alternative, and indeed it is a valid one; but at the same time, I do not see why people should not try to have their own biological child, if that is what they want. In the present book, Gab Kovacs explains in a clear and concise manner everything that one would like to know about fertility and the causes of infertility: how conception occurs and why pregnancy does not always happen; what options are available when the male partner is not fertile; how many different causes can affect the fertility of the female partner; what unexplained (idiopathic) infertility is; and what in vitro fertilization is and what it entails. This is a comprehensive and comprehensible book that provides you with all that you would like to know about human fertility, and about what can be done to address problems related to it. I trust that couples dealing with fertility issues will get a better understanding after reading this book, and as the author suggests they will keep trying as long as they emotionally, financially and physically can to fulfil their dream.

Kostas Kampourakis, Series Editor

Preface

It is generally stated that one in six couples have a problem conceiving a child. Many such couples then turn to Dr Google to learn what the problem may be. While the internet has a lot of good information, it is not 'peer reviewed' and misinformation may not be distinguished from evidence-based material by the lay person.

In this book, the whole concept of what it takes to achieve a pregnancy, how to maximise chances by appropriate timing and the available treatments are explained by a clinician who has had 40 years of experience in treating couples with subfertility.

With all the publicity about in-vitro fertilisation (IVF), couples often think they are heading for this type of treatment, but there are other alternatives, which depend on the reason for failing to conceive. This book clearly explains many treatment options. Sometimes, just understanding how best to time intercourse is sufficient to achieve a pregnancy.

My aim in writing this book was to enable couples to fully understand their fertility, their options and the benefits and risks of various treatments. While I was writing it, I used the same language that I use when consulting couples; a well-tried style that they seem to understand.

I hope that, after you have read this book, you will be better equipped to make choices about treatment options, and you will truly *Understand* your *Fertility*.

Professor Gab Kovacs

1 How Conception Occurs and Why Pregnancy Does Not Always Happen

In this first chapter, we will outline the necessary steps to achieve pregnancy. These include the three primary requirements that have to be fulfilled for an embryo to be produced, and the process for that embryo to implant and grow within the womb (uterus).

Basic Fertility Factors

For a pregnancy to occur, three basic fertility factors need to be fulfilled (Figure 1.1). First, an *adequate number* of normal sperm have to be deposited in the *correct place* at the *right time*. Second, eggs (oocytes) have to be released (ovulation) (this is described in detail in Chapter 3). Third, the passages – the uterus and tubes (Fallopian tubes) – have to be open and normal to allow the transport of sperm up, eggs down and the resulting embryo (after fertilisation) down the tubes and into the uterus. It is in the uterus that the embryo can implant and pregnancy is established.

When a couple who have difficulty conceiving are being investigated, these three basic fertility factors need to be considered.

How Do We Know If Adequate Sperm Are Being Ejaculated?

The correct number of normal sperm

Sperm is the abbreviated term that can be used for both the singular and plural:spermatozoon is one sperm and spermatozoa is more than one sperm and so is plural.

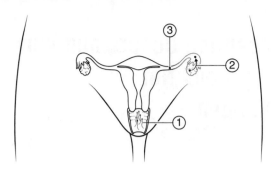

Figure 1.1 The three basic fertility factors: sperm, eggs and passages: 1. The right number of sperm in the right place at the right time, 2. Release of eggs (oocytes), and 3. The passages need to be 'normal'.

Figure 1.2 illustrates the testis and its duct system. The testis is made up of several lobules, each of which contains coiled seminiferous tubules (within which the sperm are produced), which all drain into the epididymis (the collecting duct). This then flows into the vas deferens, which is the main channel for the outflow of sperm within the semen. There are several hundred tubules in each testis. The tubules are surrounded by a capsule of fibrous tissue (tunica albuginea), which maintains their shape and structure. Within the tubules, the sperm cells mature as they progress from the base of the tubule towards the lumen. Figure 1.2 shows a cross-section of one of the tubules demonstrating sperm maturation, which continues to progress during their passage down the epididymis.

To assess the quality of sperm being ejaculated, a semen analysis is performed on an ejaculated specimen produced by masturbation (not interrupted intercourse) into a sterile pathology sample container. There are two reasons why interrupted intercourse is not suitable: First, some of the semen may be lost; second, the vaginal secretions that are acidic and harmful to the spermatozoa may contaminate the sample. Ideally, there should be 48 hours of abstinence from ejaculation prior to collecting the semen sample to be analysed. The sample should be kept at between room and body temperature until it is delivered to the laboratory, preferably within an hour. It should then be examined as soon as possible. The first assessment is the volume of semen produced (the ejaculate). The normal volume is 2–5 ml. The

A

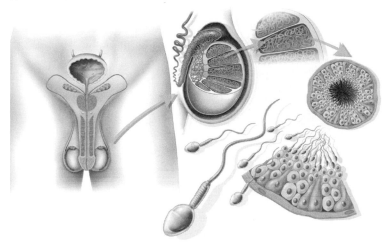

Figure 1.2 The male reproductive system. A. The testicle and its duct system. B. A single sperm as seen under the microscope.

ejaculated semen contains spermatozoa, but most of the ejaculate is composed of secretions from the accessory glands: the prostate gland and the seminal vesicles.

Next, the specimen is investigated with a special device called a Makler chamber. This is a simple-to-use device, which enables accurate sperm count and motility and morphology evaluation from an undiluted semen specimen. The Makler chamber is composed of two parts:

A lower part has a metal base and includes a flat disc made of optical flat glass. on which the sample is placed. An upper part is made up of the cover glass and is encircled by a metal ring. At the centre of the optical glass is a 1 mm grid, subdivided into 100 squares, each one measuring 0.1 × 0.1 mm. When the cover glass is placed on top, a row of 10 squares measures exactly one millionth of a millilitre (ml). Therefore, the number of sperm heads in 10 squares indicates their concentration in million per ml.

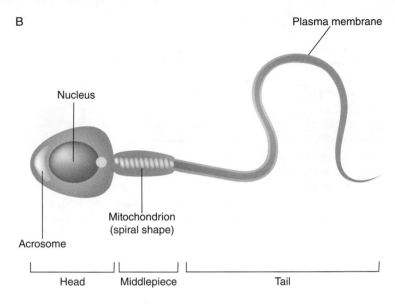

B

Plasma membrane

Nucleus

Mitochondrion (spiral shape)

Acrosome

Head   Middlepiece   Tail

Figure 1.2 (*cont.*)

The minimum concentration for a specimen to be called 'fertile' should be greater than 14 million sperm per ml. Anything less than this is called oligospermia.

The next parameter assessed is the percentage of sperm that are moving (motility) and this should be at least 40%.

The final parameter is the assessment of sperm shapes (morphology). This has to be done on a dried specimen on a glass microscope slide, treated with special dye and assessed under the microscope. Like people, sperm come in all shapes and sizes. To be considered a 'normal' sample, at least 4% of sperm present need to be the perfect shape in head, body and tail (Figure 1.2B). It is usual to assess at least two semen samples at least a couple of months apart.

Another factor that is assessed in specialised fertility laboratories is the presence or absence of antisperm antibodies in the seminal fluid (semen). Normally the sperm are confined to the ducts of the male reproductive system, and are not exposed to the immune system. This is called the blood–testis barrier. However, if sperm do escape due to trauma of the testicles, inflammation or surgery (most commonly a vasectomy), the immune system will produce antibodies to sperm, which it recognises as foreign material. This process is similar to developing antibodies against infective organisms. The antibodies are small enough to get across the blood–testis barrier and attack the spermatozoa in the duct system. This slows or immobilises the spermatozoa, impeding their ability to swim up the passages after ejaculation in the vagina. To understand this, imagine the sperm as swimmers doing laps in a pool and the antibodies as a group of playful children who jump into the pool and grab the arms and legs of the swimmers. Some of the swimmers can still complete their laps, but fewer will do so, and at a slower rate. Consequently, the presence of antisperm antibodies can be a barrier to conception.

In the correct place

It is important that sperm are deposited high into the vagina so that sperm quickly migrate into the neck (cervix) of the uterus.

This is important because the vaginal secretions are acidic and so are toxic to sperm. Once the sperm are within the cervix, they are protected from acidity by the cervical mucus and can survive for several days. Although pregnancies have resulted from sperm being ejaculated at the opening of the vagina, without vaginal penetration, the chance of conceiving is far higher if the ejaculation is high into the vagina.

Assessment of adequate technique can be obtained by asking about coital (sexual intercourse) technique such as the adequacy of erections, the sensation of ejaculation for the man and how the ejaculate feels to the woman in the vagina. This reassures the couple that ejaculation has taken place into the vagina. It is normal for some of the ejaculate to ooze out of the vagina when the woman moves, but this does not prevent conception. Some of the ejaculated sperm enter the cervical mucus within seconds, and these are the ones that will be responsible for fertilisation. Coital technique is not important unless the penis is totally misplaced or has structural abnormalities such as an opening under the shaft rather than its tip (hypospadias).

It is also possible (although rarely done) to examine the cervical mucus under the microscope after intercourse and confirm that there are sperm in the specimen. This is called a postcoital test (also known as the Sims-Huhner test, which is discussed in more detail in Chapter 5). However, this test is rarely done these days.

At the right time

The released oocyte can only be fertilised for a few hours after ovulation, so the best time for intercourse is just before ovulation. Sperm ejaculated into the vagina and protected by cervical mucus can live for a few days. They are then released in batches to travel up the passages, and may encounter an oocyte that is ready to be fertilised. It is therefore important that sperm are deposited in the vagina every couple of days around the time of ovulation. As such, couples are advised have intercourse at least every second day over the fertile week, which is described later in this chapter. There is no benefit in more frequent intercourse, and in fact some men may have difficulty building up adequate numbers of fertile sperm with more frequent ejaculations. As couples may have difficulty remembering when they have had intercourse, it can be recorded on a temperature chart (discussed in Chapter 3).

There are many myths about timing intercourse to predetermine whether a boy or girl will be conceived, including special diets and intercourse positions and restricting timing to a specific day with respect to ovulation, popularised by Dr Landrum Shettles in America in the 1960s. There is no scientific basis for these, nor any evidence that they work.

Eggs Have to Be Produced: The Basics of Ovulation

The most obvious indication of ovulation is the presence of *regular* menstrual cycles of between 25 and 32 days in duration when counting from day one of one bleed to day one of the next bleed; the start of the next cycle.

Normal menstruation lasts up to seven days, without passing clots or flooding.

Ovulation usually occurs about 14 days before the next period (menstruation, or menses), and, in regular cycles, that is between day 11 and day 18 after the start of menstruation (the fertile week). This is the time when intercourse should take place at least every second day to maximise the chance of conception. Women who have irregular and longer cycles are either not ovulating or are ovulating irregularly, and need hormonal stimulation (ovulation induction [OI]) to regulate ovulation and improve the chance of becoming pregnant (see Chapter 3). After ovulation, the released oocyte enters the outer end of the Fallopian tube, called the ampulla, where it is surrounded by sperm (see Figure 1.3). Millions of sperm are deposited into the vagina. Hundreds of thousands of these will pass through the cervix, a few thousand will enter the Fallopian tubes and a few hundred will eventually reach the oocyte in the ampulla. Only one of these will enter the oocyte to fertilise it. When a sperm penetrates the oocyte, the oocyte's shell prevents any further sperm entering.

After sperm-penetration fertilisation occurs, an early embryo develops. Both oocytes and sperm have 23 chromosomes each: one copy each of numbers

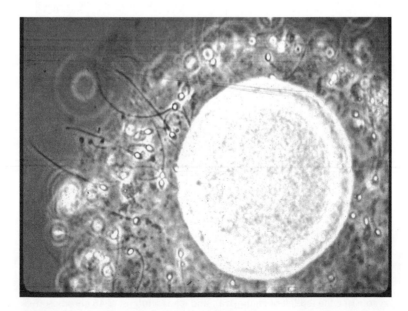

Figure 1.3 An ooocyte surrounded by many sperm.

1–22, with the oocyte only ever having X chromosomes, and the sperm having either an X or Y chromosome as its twenty-third. If the fertilised embryo has an XY complement, it will produce a male child, whereas if it has two X chromosomes (XX), the child will be female. If the oocyte has not closed its shell after a sperm has penetrated it, and a second sperm enters (polyspermy), the embryo will have 69 chromosomes, which is not compatible with life.

Fertilisation

Fertilisation requires the joining of the sperm and the oocyte, which takes place in the ampulla of the Fallopian tube.

There are four stages of the fertilisation process.

First, the sperm has to be activated. At ejaculation, sperm are not capable of fertilising an oocyte. It is only after mixing with vaginal secretions that they undergo changes, which are collectively known as capacitation, and give them the ability to bind to and penetrate the glycoprotein covering of the oocyte.

Second, the sperm (a fast-moving small cell with a head and midpiece measuring about 5 μm) has to bind to the much larger and immobile oocyte (about 100 μm in diameter). Figure 1.3 shows an oocyte surrounded by many sperm, one of which eventually binds to the oocyte as the 'chosen sperm'. The binding of the oocyte and the sperm occurs with attraction between their membranes through the thick zona pellucida (ZP) of the oocyte. The binding is made possible when receptors on the oocyte and the sperm meet. This initiates the acrosome reaction, in which the sperm releases chemicals, which can bore a hole in the ZP.

Third, the two cells have to fuse together. The tail of the sperm is immobilised and its head and body are pulled into the interior substance of the oocyte (cytoplasm). The chromosomes of the sperm are included in a new membrane envelope, forming the male pronucleus (see Figure 1.4).

Fourth, the sperm and oocyte chromosomes have to be joined together by the fusion of their covering membranes. The resultant embryo is initially called a zygote (see the top left of Figure 1.4), and it has a full set of 46 chromosomes: 22 pairs of autosomes plus either X and Y, or X and X.

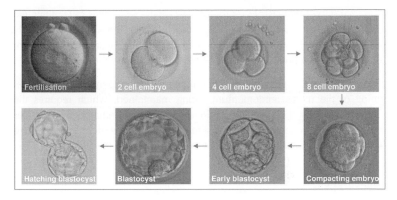

Figure 1.4 Embryo development from a fertilised oocyte to blastocyst stage.

Once the oocyte is fertilised, the ZP prevents additional sperm from penetrating. If this fails and polyspermy occurs, the zygote will have 69 chromosomes, which, as discussed earlier in this chapter, is not compatible with life.

The Passages (Uterus and Tubes) Have to Be Open and Normal

The third basic fertility factor for conception is that the tubes and uterus need to be open and 'normal' (this is discussed in detail in Chapter 4) to allow the oocyte and sperm to unite in the ampulla and then be transported to the uterine cavity. During this time, the early embryo starts to divide, comprising 4–8 cells by day three after ovulation. The cells in the embryo keep dividing as it is transported to the uterine cavity, by which time it is five days old and consists of about 100 cells (see Figure 1.4). During this rapid growth, the Fallopian tube provides nutrition until the embryo establishes its blood supply with the development of the placenta (afterbirth). As such, the Fallopian tubes are not just 'a piece of plumbing' connecting the uterus to the ovary, but complex structures responsible for transporting the sperm and oocytes (gametes), and then the embryo, and providing the only source of nutrition to the embryo for its rapid cell division and development during the four to five days it takes to reach the uterus. The lining (epithelium) of the tubes is intricate, being covered by fine hairs (cilia), which beat in a co-ordinated rhythm to sweep the sperm, oocytes and the embryo along its surface (see Figure 4.6 in Chapter 4).

The final part of the passages is the uterine cavity, which has to facilitate the implantation of the developing embryo, helping it to establish its blood supply via the early placenta. The presence of inflammation, scarring or polyps or fibroids in the uterine cavity could all prevent this.

The survival and implantation of the early embryo is dependent on the inner lining of the uterus (endometrium) being maintained, which requires the corpus luteum in the ovary to continue secreting the female sex hormones oestrogen and progesterone, which stimulate the endometrium to be retained until the placenta takes over at about three months into the pregnancy.

Implantation

Successful implantation requires a healthy blastocyst, a receptive endometrium and effective communication between the two.

The endometrium is only receptive for a few days – called the window of implantation – after which implantation is not possible.

When the developing embryo is about five days old and has multiplied to about 100 cells, it reaches what is called the blastocyst stage (see Figure 1.4), which is when it attaches to the endometrium, and the epithelium secretes a number of biochemical substances (called enzymes), which are important for implantation. The endometrium of the uterine develops protrusions called pinopodes, which help the blastocyst adhere to the endometrial lining. The attachment of the blastocyst is enhanced by the enzymes that are secreted by the endometrium, and a pathway for absorbing nutrients is established as the early placenta. During this time, the rapidly dividing cells of the blastocyst divide into two distinct layers called the cytotrophoblasts and the syncytiotrophoblasts. The inner layer (cytotrophoblasts) will form the embryo, while the outer layer (syncytiotrophoblasts) will form the placenta and membranes surrounding the fetus.

A successful pregnancy requires that the endometrial tissue have sufficient exposure to progesterone to support the endometrial lining and prevent expulsion of the trophoblasts. The syncitiotrophoblast cells secrete a hormone called human chorionic gonadotrophin (HCG). HCG acts as a message to the corpus luteum to keep it functioning, enabling the continued production of progesterone. Until the placenta fully develops after two to three months, the corpus luteum is the source of progesterone and oestrogen for the developing pregnancy. The hormones stimulate the cells of the endometrium to accumulate nutrients and the development of blood vessels to support the blastocyst. As fetal blood vessels develop, the mother's uterine arteries develop spiral arterioles, which form the feto-maternal circulation, which allows nutrients and waste through.

Finally, rather than passively accepting the attaching embryo, the endometrium appears to play an active role in blastocyst selection. This is evident by abnormal embryos triggering a chemical signal within the endometrium, which then has the ability to respond to that signal by engulfing the blastocyst and destroying it.

Age and Conceiving

A woman's fertility gradually declines in her thirties, particularly after age 35 (see Figure 1.5). At peak fertility, a healthy, fertile woman has a 25% chance of conceiving each month when she has well-timed intercourse with a fertile man.

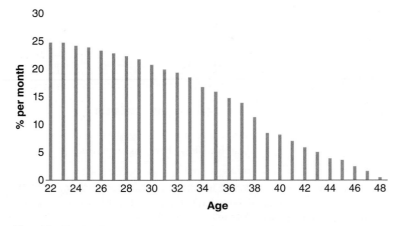

The Age Factor
The average chance of natural conception per month

Figure 1.5   The Age Factor.

By age 40, a woman's chance of conception is less than 5% per menstrual cycle, which means that fewer than 5 out of every 100 women are successful after each month of trying to conceive.

Women do not remain fertile until the menopause. Most women become unable to have a successful pregnancy some time in their mid-forties, although they may continue to menstruate. This is not only due to the number of oocytes available but the quality of oocytes also gradually declines. As women age, there are more oocytes with abnormal chromosomes, but even those that are normal chromosomally have lower energy with fewer mitochondria (which are the power generators of the oocytes) and therefore are less likely to produce healthy embryos. Although couples believe that they can use fertility treatments such as in vitro fertilisation (IVF), a woman's age also affects the success rates of infertility treatments, with success declining with age.

When and How to Get Help

Most couples who want to conceive do so within 12 months of unprotected regular intercourse. So, if a couple have not conceived after a year, it is time to get some expert advice. Women in their mid-thirties or older are recommended to do so after six months of trying to conceive. The first point of call should be the family doctor or general practitioner (GP). The GP should obtain a history, organise some early investigations and treat the consultation as 'pre-pregnancy counselling' with regards to advice about diet, alcohol, smoking and weight. Blood tests ensuring that immunity to German measles (rubella) and chickenpox (varicella) is present. The GP should then refer the couple to a specialist.

A Systematic Approach to Investigations and Treatment

To advocate a logical and systematic approach to investigating and treating a couple with subfertility, an algorithm (flow chart) has been developed by the author (see Figure 1.6).

The crux is that virtually anyone can conceive these days by using IVF, OI, egg or sperm donation, or surrogacy: often referred to collectively as assisted reproductive technology (ART).

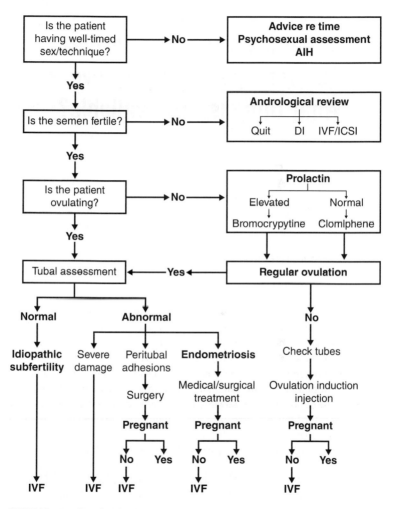

FIGURE 1.6 An algorithm for the management of a couple with subfertility.

2   Is the Male Partner Fertile? Can His Sperm be Improved? What Options Are Available?

How Are Sperm Made?

As one of the three basic fertility factors is that the 'right number of fertile sperm should be deposited into the vagina', investigating the male partner's semen quality is important and is one of the first investigations when a couple have a fertility problem. In fact, one-third of cases of subfertility are thought to be due to a male factor.

Sperm are produced within the seminiferous tubules in the testicles (see Figure 1.2A). The testis is made up of several lobules, each of which contains coiled seminiferous tubules. There are several hundred seminiferous tubules in each testis, which drain into common tributaries, and finally end up in a common collecting channel, which then flows into the vas deferens. The vas deferens carries the sperm to the urethra, which then passes through the penis, allowing an outflow during ejaculation. The immature sperm cells are produced in the periphery of the seminiferous tubules, and, as they progress into the centre of the lumen, they mature. The seminiferous tubules constitute 97% of the volume of each testicle. The other 3% is made up of interstitial cells, which are responsible for production of the hormone testosterone; the male hormone that is responsible for hair growth (especially on the chin), sex drive (libido) and muscle strength. The lobules are covered in a capsule of fibrous tissue (tunica albuginea), which maintains its shape and structure. The final maturation of sperm takes place during their travel along the seminiferous tubules, epididymis and the vas deferens, and the overall maturation process takes about 10 weeks.

The hormone that stimulates sperm production is called follicle stimulating hormone (FSH); a hormone that is secreted into the blood stream by a small gland (pituitary gland) in the brain; just behind the nose. In the female, FSH is responsible for oocyte development, and this is described in detail in Chapter 3. The second hormone that is secreted by the pituitary gland is luteinising hormone (LH). In the female, LH is responsible for triggering the release of the oocyte from the follicle (see Chapter 3), while in the male, LH stimulates the interstitial cells to secrete testosterone. Thus, there are two compartments in the testes: one that produces the gametes (sperm), and one that produces steroid hormones (androgens). Semen is made up of sperm from the testes and secretions from the prostate gland and the seminal vesicles.

What Is a Potentially Fertile Sperm Count?

The semen analysis technique was described in Chapter 1. The normal values for a semen analysis are summarised in Table 2.1. It must be remembered that there are significant variations in semen analyses performed on different days. Therefore, it is recommended that at least two samples are examined, separated by a couple of months, as sperm production takes three months.

One abnormal parameter on its own is not a predictor of infertility, but multiple abnormalities are more significant.

In andrology (the study of male fertility) laboratories, semen is often tested for antisperm antibodies, the presence of which is a significant abnormal finding.

Semen analysis	Minimum values
Volume	1.5 ml
Sperm concentration	15 million per ml
Sperm motility	40%
Sperm morphology	4% normal forms
Number of white blood cells	Less than 1 million/ml

Table 2.1 Minimum values for a semen analysis to be called normal (World Health Organization; WHO)

Clinical Assessment

Although attention is often first focused on semen analysis, the male partner should be treated as a patient and the regimen of history, examination and then investigations should be followed.

History-taking should question about age of puberty, undescended testes, trauma or torsion of testicles, infections (especially mumps), hair growth and sex drive. A history of chest infections may suggest cystic fibrosis. This is an inherited condition, which affects the mucus-secreting cells in the lungs and is often associated with congenital absence of the vasa deferentia, resulting in obstruction. As no sperm can get through, there is no sperm in the ejaculate (azoospermia). It is also important to identify any medication that may affect sperm production, especially any hormone preparations such as androgens used by bodybuilders, or chemotherapy used for treating cancers or other conditions such as arthritis. Alcohol, smoking and recreational drug use should be asked about.

Examination should include a general examination, recording of height and weight, examination of the scrotum for size of testes (expressed as volume in cubic centimetres and assessed by comparing their size to samples on a bead orchidometer – see Figure 2.1) and dilated veins around the testes (varicocele), and palpating the vasa deferentia, confirming that there is a vas deferens present on each side.

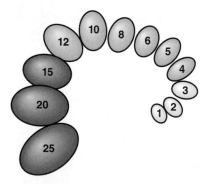

Figure 2.1 An orchidometer, used to measure testes by comparison.

Special tests include measuring hormone levels and ultrasound scan of the scrotum.

Which Hormones Should Be Measured?

In a male with a subnormal semen analysis, FSH, LH and testosterone should be measured. Most andrologists (hormone specialists who treat male fertility) also measure the hormone prolactin and undertake thyroid function tests as abnormal levels of these hormones can also affect sperm production.

Genetic Tests

In men with azoospermia or severe oligospermia (less than 5 million/ml) testing their chromosome makeup (karyotype) is recommended. Klinefelter syndrome – a condition caused by an extra X sex chromosome (resulting in XXY chromosome makeup – affects about 1 in 650 newborn boys and is among the most common sex-chromosome disorders. It has also been recognised that men with azoospermia or significant oligospermia may have small segments of their Y chromosome missing (microdeletion), which is diagnosed by extracting DNA from white blood cells from a man's blood sample, and then analyse it.

What Causes a Subnormal Semen Quality?

A man who produces no sperm (azoospermia) is called azoospermic. If there are sperm present but reduced numbers, this is called oligospermia. When the sperm movement is reduced (reduced motility) this is called asthenospermia.

Sperm shape or morphology is complicated. Just like people, sperm come in all shapes and sizes. A 'normal' sperm has an oval head with a long tail (see Figure 1.2B). Abnormal sperm have a misshapen or large or small head, or a misshapen crooked or double tail. Typically, only 4–10% of sperm in a semen sample have 'normal' morphology, so that the majority look abnormal under the microscope. Having abnormal shape may affect a sperm's ability to progress and reach the oocyte, or to fertilise it. Abnormal morphology is probably only a factor in preventing pregnancy if nearly 100% of the sperm are affected. The various shapes of sperm seen in an ejaculate are shown in Figure 2.2

Type

Normal forms

Amorphous

Megalo

Small

Elongated

Duplicated

Immature

Loose

Midpiece
abnormality

Cytoplasmic
droplets

Coiled tails

Multiple tails

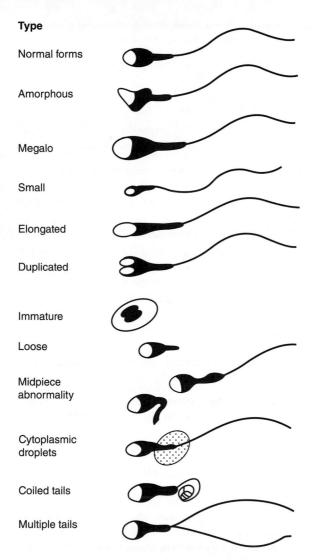

Figure 2.2 Different shapes of sperm, showing possible abnormalities.

In many men with abnormal semen analysis, there is no readily identifiable cause. However, there are a number of recognised reasons:

- Lack of sperm production due to inadequate hormonal stimulus where insufficient amounts of FSH are produced: This is called pre-testicular azoospermia.
- The seminiferous tubules being unable to produce sperm (this is called testicular azoospermia): Causes include undescended testes, previous torsion of a testicle, injury or inflammation of the testis, damage caused by drugs such as cancer treatments (chemotherapy), genetic causes (Klinefelter syndrome or Y chromosome deletions) and very often 'unknown' (idiopathic) causes.
- Obstruction to sperm outflow: Obstruction of the ducts. This is called obstructive azoospermia.
- Disorders of the accessory glands (prostate or seminal vesicles).

One of the commonest causes of seminiferous tubule failure is undescended testicles; a condition in which one or both testicles do not migrate into the scrotum. Another frequent cause is mumps infection, especially if the infection was contracted after puberty. Other causes include inflammation due to infection, or the effect of injury (e.g. torsion of the testicle). Some chemicals and drugs can also damage the seminiferous tubules. The most severe are cytotoxic drugs and X-ray therapy, which are used in treating cancer. The effect of these causes of testicular failure mean that the 'sperm factory' does not work.

The second group of causes is when the sperm delivery system is blocked, either within the seminiferous tubules or in the major outflow channels: the epididymis or vas deferens. This could be an inherited cause where the vasa deferentia have not developed a lumen and are blocked, or due to a previous vasectomy. Some sexually transmitted infections, such as gonorrhoea, can also cause scarring and blockage of duct system.

Can a Subnormal Sperm Count Be Treated?

First, having a subnormal semen analysis does not mean that a man is infertile. It may just mean that conception will take longer. General health measures should be recommended, such as reducing weight in obese men, having a good diet, abstaining from cigarettes, minimising alcohol intake and avoiding any recreational drugs. The treatment of any medical conditions (e.g. diabetes) should be optimised.

There are a few causes of subnormal sperm count that can be treated. A rare but easily treatable pre-testicular cause is when the pituitary gland does not produce FSH hormone. The condition is called hypogonadotropic hypogonadism. As in women (Chapter 3), replacing FSH by injections of FSH hormone preparation will stimulate sperm production and restore male fertility. Often, pretreatment with HCG hormone (which is biochemically equivalent to LH) is tried initially, and this may restore sperm production. If thyroid function is abnormal, or prolactin is elevated, these should be normalised with treatment.

If the number of white blood cells in the semen are elevated, especially if IVF is contemplated, a course of antibiotics should be considered as this is a sign of infection and may interfere with fertilisation.

Men with antisperm antibodies used to be treated with immunosuppression using drugs that suppress the immune system (high-dose corticosteroids). While this was sometimes successful, the side effects can be severe, and the use of IVF with microinjection (intracytoplasmic sperm injection) (see Chapter 6 and Figure 2.3) has superseded this treatment.

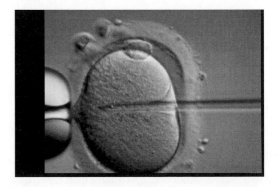

Figure 2.3   Intracytoplasmic sperm injection (ICSI). A fine glass pipette is used to inject a single sperm into the substance (cytoplasm) of the oocyte.

Surgical treatment is sometimes possible. However, often the blockage is in the small ducts of the epididymis and surgery is not possible. At the other extreme, the blockage may be in the vas deferens, such as after a vasectomy. Surgery for blockage of the vas deferens can be performed using microsurgery – vasectomy reversal – and is quite successful. However, the chance of successful pregnancy after rejoining a blocked vas deferens is significantly decreased if there are antisperm antibodies present in the bloodstream. Using IVF with ICSI is the back-up option.

A controversial treatment is surgery on the dilated veins (varicose veins) around the testes (varicoceles). Although varicoceles are also common in men with normal semen analysis, it is suggested that they can interfere with sperm production due to increased temperature or decreased oxygen supply to the seminiferous tubules. The treatment offered is to tie off these dilated veins: about two-thirds of men improve their sperm numbers or motility after surgery, and some achieve pregnancies. Further research is needed to explain how varicoceles affect sperm production, and to identify which men may be helped by ligation of their varicocele.

Unfortunately for most men with a subfertile semen analysis, there is no cause identified. Consequently, there is no effective treatment, and IVF with or without ICSI is their best option. Unfortunately, many possible remedies have been suggested and prescribed, including vitamins and herbs, but all are unproven. Many are thought to be as effective as 'snake oil' and they are not recommended.

Artificial Insemination with Partner's Semen

Artificial insemination with partner's semen was historically known as artificial insemination with husband (AIH). If the cause of the subfertility is a mechanical problem such as inability to maintain an erection, penile abnormality, vaginal spasm (vaginismus) limiting penetration by the penis or retrograde ejaculation (where the semen passes into the bladder rather than out through the urethra), then collecting a masturbated specimen, or sperm recovered from the bladder, and artificially inseminating it into the partner's cervix has a very high success rate. Artificial insemination can be either done blindly by the woman or her partner, or by direct visualisation of the cervix by a nurse or doctor.

For blind insemination, the semen can be injected by a syringe and plastic cannula or an instrument like a turkey baster into the vagina. However, it is more efficient to inject directly into the cervix. This requires the insertion of a vaginal speculum, such as used for taking smear tests, and, when the cervix is visualised, the semen is injected under vision into the cervical canal. Sometimes intrauterine insemination is undertaken by passing a fine cannula through the cervical canal and injecting the semen into the uterine cavity. For intrauterine AIH to be undertaken, the semen must be specially prepared and some of the chemicals within removed.

In cases of decreased sperm numbers, decreased motility or few normal-shaped sperm, the use of AIH is more controversial. This is sometimes performed, and it requires having the semen sample specially prepared to obtain a most fertile subsample for insemination. This subsample is prepared by selecting the most motile sperm or concentrating the sperm within a smaller volume of seminal fluid. To further improve the chance of pregnancy, the female is often stimulated with fertility hormones to produce two or three oocytes. Although this treatment is sometimes successful and is less complicated and cheaper than IVF, it has a lower success rate than IVF (about 10–15% per cycle) and has the risk of producing multiple pregnancies if several oocytes ovulate.

How Does IVF Technology Help?

Although IVF was developed to overcome infertility for women with damaged Fallopian tubes, the number of sperm required to fertilise oocytes in the test tube (in vitro) is only tens of thousands. The hypothesis was therefore suggested that men who did not have enough sperm to fertilise their partners' oocytes through intercourse may be able to do so by IVF. When the hypothesis was put to the test, it became apparent that this was so, and the use of IVF for the treatment of male-factor subfertility became standard practice. Subsequently, the number of sperm required was further reduced by inseminating oocytes in small drops of culture medium (microdrops), and ultimately by using microinjection when only a single sperm is injected into each oocyte: ICSI (see Figure 2.3). Thus, men with very few sperm in their ejaculate can now become fathers.

Even men who have no sperm in their ejaculate can sometimes use IVF technology. This is easily possible for men who have obstructive azoospermia as techniques have been developed where, after injecting a local anaesthetic, a fine needle can be passed through the scrotum into the obstructed duct system and mature sperm can be aspirated. This is particularly easy after vasectomy where the obstructed distended vas deferens can be palpated, but it is also suitable for small duct obstruction where the needle is just inserted into the testicular tissue, hoping to blindly recover some sperm. Specimens of sperm obtained by this technique are only suitable for use by microinjection and IVF.

The next major breakthrough is for men with testicular azoospermia. Although they do not have detectable sperm in their ejaculate, these men sometimes still have small areas of sperm production in their testicles. It may be possible under a general anaesthetic, with the testicle surgically opened and using an operating microscope, to identify some functioning seminiferous tubules, which can be seen distended with microscopic magnification. If these tubules are then opened using microsurgical instruments, some sperm may be harvested, which then can be used for IVF, again with microinjection. These can either be used fresh or frozen and then thawed when the man's partner's oocytes have been harvested.

The techniques used for IVF are discussed in detail in Chapter 6.

Sperm Donation

Although most men with oligospermia and some with azoospermia can become fathers using IVF technology, there will always be some for whom the techniques don't work, or who do not wish to use IVF. An alternative for these couples is to use sperm donation: replacing their sperm with that from a fertile donor; a practice that has been used for many decades. Initially, practitioners would recruit a man to masturbate and take his fresh specimen of semen to the clinic on the day that the prospective recipient (whose partner was infertile) was expected to be on her estimated fertile day. The semen was then injected into her vagina using a speculum and syringe, aiming for the cervix, and that was all that was to the process. There was no possibility of matching, nor was the semen screened for quality, and the donor was unscreened for heritable disease and infections. The doctors' record-keeping was variable, and no official records of paternity were kept. Nevertheless, the infertile couple would achieve their aim of having a baby, although it may have taken several tries.

The use of donor insemination (DI) has become more refined during the last 50 years when sperm freezing and banking was developed. This technique was developed for animal husbandry, and the medical profession simply copied what was done in the dairy industry. In fact, the equipment initially used was purchased from veterinary suppliers. With current sperm banking, the ejaculated sperm is mixed with a glycerol and egg-yolk preservation medium, which protects the sperm from damage during freezing. The specimens are then frozen in small straws and stored in liquid nitrogen at $-196°C$. Once frozen, the specimens can be kept frozen indefinitely. When the particular specimen is required for use, it is removed from the liquid-nitrogen storage tank and allowed to thaw at room temperature over a few minutes. It is then ready to be inseminated into the matched recipient. Many countries have a limit on how long sperm can be frozen (10 years is usual) as there is concern about intergenerational reproduction. Some ethicists are concerned about the possibility that sperm stored for decades could be used to inseminate offspring several generations down the line, even after the donor has long deceased, which they consider undesirable.

How Does Sperm Donation Work?

Terminology
The person who donates the semen is the sperm donor. He becomes the genetic father of any child/children born. The woman who is inseminated is the recipient and becomes the genetic mother (her oocyte), the birth mother (as she gives birth to the child) and continues as the social mother as she is responsible for the child's upbringing. The partner of the woman who is inseminated is not the genetic father, but he is the birth father (as he supports his partner during the process) and social father as he is also responsible for the child's upbringing. If the donor has his own partner/wife, their consent is usually required for the donation.

Who Can Donate Sperm?
Any man who offers to be a sperm donor is first screened for medical and family history. Donors will not be accepted if they suffer from an illness, disease or genetic condition that poses an unacceptable risk of being passed on to any child conceived from the donation. Most clinics restrict donors to under 40–45 years of age as there is some suggestion that chromosomal

abnormalities are more common from older fathers. If there is no medical reason to prevent donation, a specimen of semen is examined to ensure that they are potentially fertile.

How Are Donors Screened?

A 'test freeze' is performed to ensure the donor's semen freezes and thaws with a good survival rate. Next, the donor is usually examined, and a blood test is taken to determine their blood group (for matching purposes) and to exclude infections by looking for antibodies that may herald these. All clinics screen for syphilis (although this is quite rare in the community, it can be disastrous for any baby conceived), hepatitis and HIV, while some clinics screen for cytomegalovirus (CMV). Because some infections, especially HIV, may take a few weeks to produce antibodies in the blood, which is what provides a warning that the donor is infected, there is an incubation period, or 'window', where a person may be infectious but not yet identifiable as infected. For this reason, the semen collected for banking is placed in quarantine for a few months and the potential donor is asked to return for a blood test, which has to be negative, before the sample is released for selection from the sperm bank. Using this quarantine period virtually eliminates the risk of transmission of these infectious diseases.

Counselling and Legal Status

Sperm donors and their partners are counselled to make sure they understand that they are donating sperm that will result in children being born. They also need to understand the legal situation. Most countries have passed legislation that states the donor has no legal rights to any offspring produced, and that the children have no legal recall on the donor. In many countries, the donors must be willing to have their identity revealed to any offspring. In many countries, including the UK since 2005, anyone conceived with the help of a donor can ask for their donor's name, date of birth and last known address when they turn 18 years of age. Not all offspring will ask for their donor's details or decide to contact them. There is no obligation to have contact, but some children do wish to meet their donor.

Recipient couples have been counselled to be honest with the children born from sperm donation, and, as soon as the children are old enough, to explain that they were conceived from a sperm donation. It was suggested that they explain that 'Dad' was unable to make sperm and a kind man donated sperm to enable Mum and Dad to have children. Julia Paul, a counsellor from Sydney produced a book with illustrations in 1988 to help parents achieve this. Nevertheless, the author and colleagues' research showed that two out of three parents kept the mode of conception secret. We studied the functioning of families with primary school-age children conceived using anonymous donor sperm. We wanted to know how families with children conceived using donor sperm function as the children grow up. The study was an observational study comparing 63 DI families with 987 'couple' families, 364 'single-mother' families and 112 'stepfather' families as part of the Australian Institute of Family Studies Children and Family Life (CFL) study. CFL involved the collection of data on family functioning and child well-being from all resident parents: a family and child questionnaire for the 'primary' parent (FACQ-P1) and a family relationship questionnaire for the 'other' parent (FRQ-P2).

We found that families with children aged 5–12 years conceived through anonymous donor sperm were functioning well when compared to other family types with children of the same developmental stage. This study further reassures us that families conceived with anonymous donor sperm do not function any differently from other family types.

Although sociologists suggest that keeping secrets within a family may affect relationships, our studies found that families where the use of donor sperm for the children's conception was secret functioned as well as families where children were told about their biological origins. Today, with the availability of affordable and easily accessible genetic testing, it is impossible keep genetic identity secret, and couples are strongly recommended not to keep the use of gamete donation secret.

With the removal of anonymity, many children have actually met their donors: some were very happy stories, but others have not had a happy ending. Children conceived from donor sperm have also met half-siblings.

When sperm banking commenced in the late 1970s, donors were promised that their donation would always anonymous. In most countries, the removal of anonymity was prospective; that is, from a certain date, prospective donors were warned that their identity would be released to any offspring, when the child reached 18 years of age. However, in the state of Victoria, Australia, despite strong opposition from health-care providers, the parliament passed a law in 2017, removing anonymity retrospectively, so that donors who had donated on the understanding that they would always be anonymous were suddenly in a position where their genetic children could contact them. There was no compulsion on any meetings, but even contact by telephone or mail could be embarrassing if the donors' partners were not aware of the history of sperm donation.

Although it is only a minority of offspring who wish to find their donor, some are very much obsessed by this need. In the author's experience, this is often offspring from families where the social parents have separated.

Reimbursement

In most countries, donors can be paid a small amount of £20–40 per donation to cover their expenses for attending the clinic. They are not paid for the semen as trafficking in human tissue is not acceptable, and the semen is a true donation. This is different in the United States where sperm and egg banking are commercial processes, and the males who provide semen are sperm vendors.

How Is the Sperm Matched?

When DI was done informally, there was no matching; sperm was just used from any member of the donor panel who was available to produce a sample on the required day. After sperm banking was introduced, it was still within an air of secrecy, and there was a desire to make the child appear to be that of his or her social father, so the donor's blood group and physical characteristics (race, complexion, height, build and hair and eye colour) were matched to resemble that of the social father. Although secrecy is now unrealistic because of the access to cheap genetic testing such as Ancestry DNA®, it is still usual to match the blood group and physical characteristics of the donor to the partner of the recipient (the social father). Physical characteristics are matched so the child's are compatible with those of his or her social father, although genetics is sometimes unpredictable.

It is desirable to use a donor who has a rhesus (Rh) negative blood group if the recipient (mother) is Rh negative to prevent Rh immunisation during the pregnancy. Rh is a minor blood group factor, with 85% of people being Rh positive. The potential problem is that, if an Rh-negative woman (15% of population) conceives with an Rh-positive man, the baby may be Rh positive. If some of the baby's Rh-positive red blood cells enter the mother's circulation (which usually occurs at delivery but sometimes during pregnancy) her immune system will make anti-Rh antibodies (similar to the mechanism for antisperm antibodies as described above). These Rh antibodies are small enough to cross the placenta and attack the red blood cells of an Rh-positive baby. The red cells are then broken down, resulting in anaemia due to a shortage of red blood cells, as well as a build-up of bilirubin(jaundice) due to the released haemoglobin (the oxygen-carrying component of red blood cells) then entering the baby's circulation.

Sometimes a 'known donor' is used, where a donor specifically donates for a particular recipient. For example, a fertile brother may donate for use by his infertile brother's partner, or a man's father donates for his infertile son. There was some opposition in the early days of DI to these unusual methods of parenting, but today they are widely accepted. Alternatively, a good friend may be asked to be the semen donor for a couple. The same process of screening and counselling is carried out for these 'known donors' as for sperm-bank donors.

The Insemination

The insemination process is quite simple. The most important step is to ascertain when the female is ovulating. This is done by detecting the rise of LH hormone – which causes ovulation – usually in a woman's urine (sometimes blood) test. As will be explained in detail in Chapter 3, ovulation occurs about 24 hours after the LH rise, and the insemination is performed at that time. For women who have irregular menstrual cycles and ovulate irregularly, OI with oral tablets or sometimes with injections of FSH is used (see Chapter 3).

The selected sperm specimen is thawed, and the semen is then inseminated on the day of expected ovulation into the female's cervix. The process causes minimal discomfort, and it is very similar to a smear test, which most women are used to. The recipient rests for a few minutes before resuming her normal activities.

Outcomes

Unfortunately, not every insemination results in conception. The success rate of DI with thawed frozen sperm is about 10–15% per cycle. In real life, couples do not plan to get pregnant in a specific month, but plan to try for several months. Similarly, after six cycles of DI, it would be expected that 50–75% of couples would be pregnant.

Once a pregnancy is achieved, it is no different to a natural pregnancy. There is the same chance of early pregnancy loss (about 10–15%) as for natural pregnancies. Using thawed frozen sperm does not increase the rate of pregnancy loss. Theoretically, as potential donors with a known family history of genetic disease are excluded, the chance of an abnormality should be even lower in children conceived with banked donor semen. For natural conceptions, the chance of having a major abnormality of the baby is about 3%, and another 3% for a minor abnormality. From follow-up studies of real-world experience, freezing and thawing sperm does not increase the risk of abnormalities at birth.

We have compared families that were formed by DI when the children were primary-school age, as described above, and, in summary, found that the family relationships were no worse than in naturally conceived families.

For several decades, couples have been advised to be honest with their children about the method of conception. Couples have been provided with non-identifying information about the donor to help them describe him to the child, and now, in many countries, the donor's identity can be obtained when the child reaches 18 years of age. However, there are many couples (two out of three in our follow-up study) who decide to keep the use of a donor secret, but in today's environment, with relatively cheap and readily available genetic testing, this is risky. There is a high chance that the offspring may find out that their social father is not their genetic father, and this could cause serious problems in their relationship. It is therefore recommended that the children are told from an early age how they were conceived.

Unfortunately, sometimes even several cycles of DI do not achieve a pregnancy, and then the option is to use IVF with donor sperm. Some couples prefer to attempt IVF with donor sperm as their first option – although it is more complicated and more expensive – because of its higher success rate (30–50% per cycle depending on the woman's age) and the shortage of donor semen.

3 Physiology of the Menstrual Cycle and Anovulation Treatment

Hormonal Control of Ovulation

The menstrual cycle is controlled by the hypothalamic-pituitary-ovarian axis (see Figure 3.1).

The pituitary gland sits at the base of the brain, behind the bridge of the nose. It is a small gland – the size of a cherry – and it is connected to the hypothalamus (the lower part of the brain) where gonadotrophin releasing hormone (GnRH), (a protein hormone made up of 10 amino acids) is secreted. The GnRH is secreted in a pulsatile manner, and it is the pattern of pulses (frequency and amplitude) that determines the response from the pituitary gland by FSH and LH secretion.

GnRH is secreted into the pituitary gland via venous channels, which then stimulates the gland to secrete FSH (the hormone responsible for stimulating the developing follicles). FSH levels in the blood are higher in the earlier part of the menstrual cycle when a new batch of follicles is stimulated to develop, then decrease during the second half of the menstrual cycle, with a small peak just prior to ovulation (in parallel with the LH rise – see next paragraph).

The second hormone secreted from the pituitary gland is LH, which should really be called the ovulating hormone as it is responsible for ovulating (releasing the mature egg from the ovarian follicle). The level of LH is low at basal (background) levels throughout the cycle, except for the LH peak, which is responsible for ovulation. This LH peak is followed by ovulation about 36 hours after it starts to rise, and 24 hours after it peaks. Elevated levels of LH can be detected for about 24 hours (see Figure 3.2).

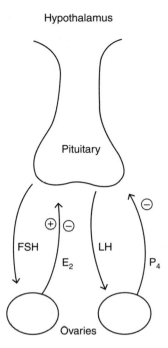

Hypothalamus

Pituitary

FSH

E_2

LH

P_4

Ovaries

Figure 3.1 Interaction within the hypothalamic-pituitary-ovarian axis. The hypothalamus stimulates the pituitary gland to secrete FSH, which stimulates follicular development. The follicle secretes the hormone oestradiol (shown as E_2 in the figure), which turns off FSH (negative feedback). When the E_2 level reaches a level that suggests the follicle is mature, the release of LH is triggered (positive feedback). This then triggers ovulation (release of the oocyte: ovulation) and progesterone is secreted from the cells that used to surround the ovum and the corpus luteum (shown as P_4 in the figure).

Development of the Ovarian (Graafian) Follicle

A woman is born with about one million potential oocytes, of which only about 400 mature (one a month for about 35 years) in her lifetime. Each month, a batch of follicles start to mature, which consist of an oocyte surrounded by a group of cells. As the follicles start to develop from day one of the cycle, the cells surrounding the egg (the granulosa cells) start to secrete the female steroid hormone, oestrogen. Oestrogen is a hormone that circulates

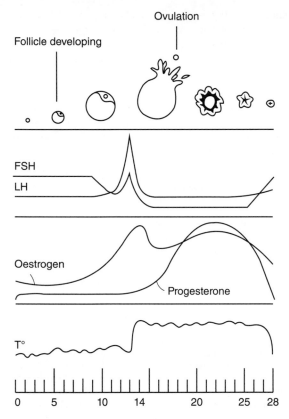

Figure 3.2 Hormonal levels during an ovulatory cycle, with associated changes in the ovarian follicle. In the early part of the cycle, FSH is higher as it needs to stimulate follicles, which secrete oestrogen, with rising levels as they grow. LH is basal thorough the cycle, except for the LH peak, which is followed by ovulation about 24 hours later. After ovulation, the shell of the follicle (corpus luteum) starts secreting progesterone as well as oestrogen. If no conception occurs, the corpus luteum succumbs, and both oestrogen and progesterone levels decline.

throughout the body and affects many organs such as the breasts, the vagina and the skin. From a fertility perspective, its most important role is to stimulate the uterine lining (endometrium) to thicken; a phenomenon called prolifer-ation. It also has the effect of regulating the pituitary gland, so that as the oestrogen level rises, FSH secretion is reduced, similar to the thermostat of a central heating system turning off the heater as the temperature rises. This is called negative feedback. This negative feedback by oestrogen on the pituitary gland ensures that FSH secretion is limited and that the stimulation to the ovary is moderated, and thus usually only one oocyte matures and is released. This becomes the leading follicle, with the other follicles degenerating (undergoing what is called atresia). Only the leading follicle (which will ovulate) matures, and that is why humans do not produce 'litters' and so 99% of natural pregnancies result in a single baby being born. If two follicles mature and two eggs are released, twins can result: these are called dizygotic twins. When a single embryo splits into two, this results in monozygotic twins, but this occurs some time after fertilisation in the uterus and is not hormonally driven.

To confuse the issue, oestrogen also has a positive feedback effect on the pituitary gland. This means that when the leading follicle reaches a diameter of about 18 mm and bulges out from the surface of the ovary and the oocyte is ready to be released, a critical level of oestrogen is reached, which signals that the follicle is mature. This stimulates the LH to be released from the pituitary gland, and the resulting LH peak in turn stimulates ovulation. This can be compared to the shell of a hen's egg cracking, with the yolk being released and passing down the Fallopian tubes, while the egg white and eggshell (theca cells) remain as the corpus luteum (yellow body in Latin: the yellow colour comes from the buildup of carotene in the thecal cells). The corpus luteum is responsible for secreting hormones that are essential for a pregnancy to be established (both oestrogen and progesterone), which stimulate the uterine lining (endometrium) to thicken in anticipation – if a sperm has fertilised the ovum – of an embryo arriving a few days later.

The second female hormone, progesterone, is only produced after ovulation, and it changes the endometrium to form several glands, become rich in glycogen and undergo what is called secretory change.

The Effect of Oestrogen and Progesterone on the Endometrium

Oestrogen and progesterone are hormones that circulate throughout the body. One of their most obvious effects is on the uterine lining, resulting in a sequence of buildup of the endometrium and then, in the absence of a pregnancy, shedding (menstruation). As described above, it is the effect of the circulating oestrogen to cause the endometrium to thicken (proliferative endometrium). The endometrium is lined by epithelium, which is folded into glands supported by fibrous tissue containing blood vessels (stroma). The thickening occurs in both the supporting tissue (stroma) and the glandular tissue. After ovulation, with the production of progesterone, the endometrium becomes secretory, containing tortuous glands with lots of glycogen, which means they can provide a welcoming, nutritional environment should an embryo arrive. If a fertilised ovum does not arrive in the uterus, the corpus luteum succumbs after about 14 days and the hormone production of both oestrogen and progesterone plumets, resulting in the endometrium coming away (menstruation), and the next cycle commences.

The Effect of Oestrogen and Progesterone on Cervical Secretions (Mucus)

The other change induced by oestrogen and progesterone that can be followed through a menstrual cycle is the change in the cervical mucus, which appears in the vagina. These secretions from the cervix change throughout an ovulatory cycle. The appearance of this mucus is determined by its salt and water content. Vaginal secretions during the initial days of the menstrual cycle are dominated by menstruation. These days are followed by a time when there is little oestrogen secretion and sparse mucus is secreted; these are called 'dry days'. As the follicle grows, the amount of oestrogen secreted increases. The oestrogen stimulates the cervix to secrete copious amounts of clear stretchy mucus, referred to as fertile mucus, which increases in quantity and quality as the oestrogen level rises. This fertile mucus is thin, clear and slippery, and it resembles egg white. It reaches its maximum quantity and its most slippery consistency just prior to ovulation about day 12–14 in a 28-day cycle, when the follicle is mature, and when the oestrogen level is maximal. This fertile mucus is easy for sperm to penetrate and signifies the best time to have intercourse to maximise the chance of conception.

The secretion of progesterone only starts at ovulation. As soon as progesterone enters the circulation, it affects the salt concentration in the mucus, and its quality changes to an infertile pattern, where it becomes thick, opaque and tacky (like glue). This rapid change in mucus from fertile to infertile signals that ovulation has taken place. Once the mucus changes to the infertile pattern, penetration by sperm is inhibited, and conception is unlikely.

These changes in cervical mucus are the basis of natural family planning, known as the Billings method, whose principal theory is to avoid intercourse when the mucus suggests fertile days.

The Corpus Luteum and Pregnancy

The corpus luteum (which corresponds to the eggshell and egg white of a hen's egg and stays behind in the ovary after ovulation) has a life span of about 14 days. In the absence of a pregnancy it then succumbs, with the result that the levels of oestrogen and progesterone decline. This results in the endometrium sloughing off as menstruation, and the start of the next cycle: the first day of bleeding being defined as 'day one' of the *next* cycle. If fertilisation occurs, the early embryo secretes the HCG hormone, which has a stimulatory effect on the corpus luteum, rescues it and maintains its hormonal function so that the levels of oestrogen and progesterone do not decline, but continue to increase. This maintains the endometrium in place and prevents the onset of the next menstrual period. It is the role of the corpus luteum to secrete adequate oestrogen and progesterone during the first three months of pregnancy, a role which is then taken over by the placenta.

Is the Woman Ovulating?

Medical diagnosis is usually divided into three parts: history, examination and investigations.

The most important factor in the woman's history is her menstrual pattern. If she has regular cycles (for example 25–32 days), it is likely that her cycles are associated with ovulation (ovulatory cycles). Further supporting evidence is if she has painful periods, especially if they are associated with premenstrual symptoms (bloating, breast tenderness, and so on). The other symptoms a woman can describe are the cyclical changes in her mucous secretions from the cervix.

On *examination* the changes in the cervical mucus can be followed, and, to further increase its sensitivity, a sample can be taken from the cervix, and, after allowing the mucus to dry on a microscope slide, it can be inspected under a microscope. When oestrogen dominates, a 'ferning' pattern is seen, which disappears after ovulation. While this is possible to do and is scientifically valid, it is rarely performed today as hormone tests (described in the next section) are easier and more reliable.

The second aspect of examination is to follow a woman's basal body temperature (BBT). This is the body temperature upon waking in the morning: the basal temperature after some hours of resting.

Consequently, the temperature should be taken every morning before getting out of bed, having a drink or even moving around, thus providing the BBT. Because progesterone is thermogenic – that is, it elevates the body temperature – the average temperature in the second half of an ovulatory cycle is about 0.3–0.5 °C higher than in the follicular or first phase. This rise results in a biphasic temperature chart (see Figure 3.3A) (meaning the second half of the cycle shows an elevated average temperature compared to the first half); in contrast to a cycle in which there is no ovulation and no rise, resulting in a monophasic temperature chart (see Figure 3.3B) with the temperatures oscillating around the same level for the whole cycle. There is often a temperature dip to coincide with ovulation. While it is not always clear, with a little practice, a temperature chart is a very useful guide as to whether a woman is ovulating, and also indicates the day when ovulation occurred.

The author's own practice is to ask couples who have failed to conceive to keep temperature charts as the first line of investigation. It is a very easy process, does not cost money, has no complications and gives a couple a better understanding of what might be going on. An elevated temperature chart for more than 15 days is also the first suggestion that conception has occurred (see Figure 3.3C). If the oocyte was fertilised, the early embryo secretes HCG, which continues the progesterone (and oestrogen) secretion from the corpus luteum, prevents the endometrium from sloughing and maintains the elevated BBT. Apps are available that can help a woman track and document her temperature during the cycle (e.g. www.Fertilityfriend.com).

Here are some instructions on how to record a temperature chart:

1.   The first morning of full menstruation is taken as day one of the cycle. Record this on the chart as X for menstruation or S for spotting.

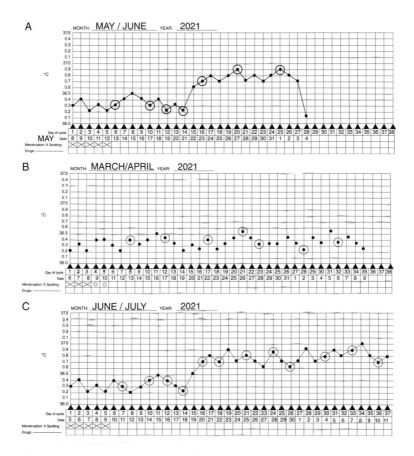

Figure 3.3   A. A biphasic temperature. The first part of the cycle has a basal level of temperature, which then elevates 0.5 °C after ovulation on day 14. B. Monophasic temperature chart. This chart shows a flat temperature with no rise, suggesting there is no ovulation. C. The temperature chart in a cycle where conception occured. Ovulation occurred on about day 14, with elevated biphasic temperature for 22 days as progesterone (and oestrogen) keep being secreted.

2. Fill in the day of the month in the space provided and record the month on the chart.
3. Use a thermometer under the tongue with a conventional thermometer, or with an infrared forehead/ear thermometer, to record basal temperature before getting out of bed, eating or moving around every morning.
4. Record the temperature on the chart by placing a dot in the appropriate square. These dots can then be joined to produce a graph.
5. The days when intercourse occurs should be recorded by putting a circle around the temperature dot.
6. Start a new chart when the next menstrual cycle starts.
7. Mark the days when medication is taken (if on OI).

Today there are investigations that are excellent indicators of whether ovulation has taken place. The most practical, and the one most commonly used, is the measurement of the progesterone level in the blood. This is easily done in a pathology laboratory using a technique called radioimmunoassay, and a result is obtained within hours. The result is usually expressed in nmol/L and most laboratories would report levels above 20 nmol/L as a level consistent with ovulation. Some laboratories still report results as ng/ml and the level suggesting ovulation varies with each one, but should be above 7 ng/ml.

Another way that ovulation can be diagnosed is by ultrasound examination of the ovaries. While this can be done on an abdominal scan through the bladder (which needs to be full of urine), it is better done through the vagina when, with appropriate manipulation and minimal discomfort, the probe can be placed next to the ovary and developing follicle(s) can be observed and measured. It is therefore possible to visualise developing follicles, which usually ovulate at about 16–20 mm in diameter, or, if the scan is performed after ovulation, it is often possible to visualise the corpus luteum as a vascular area in the ovary.

A more precise method is to perform serial scans, watching the follicle grow and then to note that it has ovulated and collapsed with the characteristic vascular changes. This of course is very time consuming and expensive and is not performed as a routine clinical method.

Another way of determining whether ovulation has taken place is to examine the endometrium under the microscope. The endometrium has to be surgically obtained, either during a small operation called dilatation and curettage (D&C), or during a procedure that can be done in the examination room called an endometrial biopsy. This requires a small cannula to be inserted through the neck of the womb and some endometrium to be 'sucked out' by using suction through the catheter. In the laboratory, the sample is soaked in a chemical called formalin – which makes the tissue solidify – then cut into thin slices, fixed on a microscope slide and stained. It can then be examined as a histological specimen and the characteristic changes of ovulation secretory changes can be diagnosed. Today, this is only done in combination with surgery if this is indicated for some other reason (see Chapter 4).

The Role of Luteinising Hormone

As described above, LH is essential for ovulation to occur, and the LH peak precedes ovulation by 24 hours. Thus, LH is a marker for when ovulation occurs, but it is *not* a test for ovulation. The LH hormone is a message from the hypothalamic-pituitary-ovarian axis to the ovarian follicle to trigger ovulation, but it does not assess whether the follicle has responded. As such, measuring LH has no place in assessing whether ovulation has taken place. It does, however, have an important role in timing when ovulation is *expected* to occur. This can be important in timing intercourse, artificial insemination or frozen embryo transfer in IVF (see Chapter 6).

Anti-Müllerian Hormone

Anti-Müllerian hormone (AMH) is a protein that is produced only by the granulosa cells surrounding the oocyte in small (primordial follicles) and medium follicles up to 8 mm in diameter. A female fetus starts secreting AMH at about 36 weeks of gestation, levels rise throughout childhood and peak in the mid-twenties, then gradually decline until undetectable levels are reached at the menopause. It has been accepted that measuring the level of AMH in the blood gives an indication of how many primordial follicles with the ability to mature in the future and ovulate are left in the ovary. AMH, therefore, has become the best available test for ovarian reserve. Age-specific AMH values have been provided by several studies. A graph showing the normal range for each age range is shown in Figure 3.4. However, the results of AMH assay, even when age specific, need to be interpreted in context of

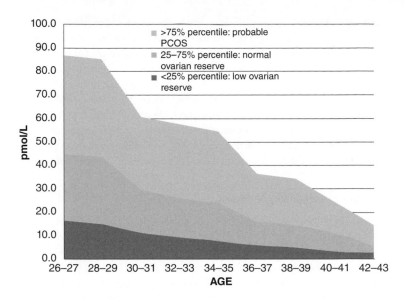

Figure 3.4 AMH level with age.

the rest of a patient's history (i.e. smoking or early onset of menopause of the woman's mother).

As AMH does give an indication of the size of the primordial follicle pool and whether a woman will go through an early menopause, it may suggest taking a more expeditious approach to her fertility treatment, especially if she wishes to conceive more than one child in the future. While AMH gives an indication of ovarian reserve, it is of no value in assessing the lack of ovulation, with the exception that very low levels of AMH associated with a lack of periods (amenorrhoea) may be indicative of premature ovarian insufficiency (POI) (previously called premature ovarian failure). This, however, is more accurately diagnosed by measuring FSH levels (see later in the chapter).

Measuring AMH level is important in determining the regimen of controlled ovarian hyperstimulation (COH), which is used for IVF. This is discussed in Chapter 6. The level of AMH has no correlation with the subsequent success of OI.

Inducing Ovulation

Before Starting

If ovulation has stopped or has become irregular, it is usually not caused by the ovaries but is the result of malfunctioning of the hormones that control ovulation. Women who do not ovulate, or who ovulate irregularly, can usually be stimulated to ovulate by OI.

It is important that women adopt a healthy lifestyle before starting treatment for absence of ovulation (anovulation). They should not smoke nor take recreational drugs, and, if overweight, they should undergo weight reduction. In some overweight women who do not ovulate, losing weight is sometimes sufficient to resume ovulation, particularly in women with polycystic ovary syndrome (PCOS), discussed later in the chapter. Other common causes of amenorrhoea are excessive weight and excessive exercise, sometimes in combination. For such women, restoring body weight to a healthy weight is also often sufficient to solve the problem. Stress and general ill health can also inhibit ovulation.

Before commencing OI, a number of investigations should be carried out. Hormone profile for FSH, LH, prolactin and thyroid stimulating hormone (TSH) should be measured. Immunity to German measles (rubella), and chickenpox (varicella), should be confirmed as women should be immune or be immunised for these infections before becoming pregnant. It is also important that male partner's semen analysis is checked before commencing OI.

Elevated Prolactin

Elevated prolactin (hyperprolactinaemia) inhibits ovulation. Symptoms may include a leakage of milky secretions from the breasts (galactorrhoea) and sometimes headache. Anxiety and stress (even the stress of a blood test) can elevate prolactin levels slightly. Other causes of raised prolactin include underactive thyroid or adrenal gland, and liver disease. Certain medicines, such as blood-pressure treatment and psychiatric medications like tranquilisers, may elevate prolactin. If prolactin level is elevated to more than twice the upper limit of normal, then the possibility of a non-cancerous tumour (pituitary adenoma) of the pituitary gland needs to be excluded. This is done by requesting a medical imaging technique called a CT scan. While these pituitary adenomas are not cancer and do not spread, they can expand and put pressure on the nerves to the eyes and cause visual disturbance. Fortunately, they are very rare, but they do inhibit ovulation.

Once excluded, the elevated prolactin can be normalised by oral tablets (bromocriptine or cabergoline). When the prolactin level returns to normal, ovulation usually recommences spontaneously.

Possible side effects of bromocriptine may include nausea, constipation, headaches, nasal congestion and dizziness.

If Prolactin Is Normal, First Exclude Ovarian Failure

If the prolactin level is normal, it is important to ensure that FSH level is not elevated. As described earlier in this chapter, FSH stimulates follicles to grow, with the level of FSH being suppressed by oestrogen secreted from growing follicles (negative feedback). If there is no follicular response and no oestrogen being secreted, the FSH level will persistently be very elevated (greater than 25 mIU/mL). Remember, prior to ovulation there is a temporary rise in FSH along with the LH rise, but this peak is never above 25 mIU/mL. Elevated FSH is normal for women who have gone through the menopause and have run out of potential follicles, but if it happens in a woman under 40 years of age, it is called premature menopause, or POI. Such women have small ovaries and have very low levels of oestrogen, and they can experience symptoms of the menopause such as hot flushes, dry vagina and lack of libido.

Often, there is no explanation for POI, but it can be caused by chromosomal abnormalities, immunological disorders and, very rarely, iron or sugar-storage disorders. There may be a similar history in their mothers. However, in many instances there is no cause identified, and so it is called 'idiopathic'. As the principle of OI is to increase FSH levels and thus induce ovulation, women with POI cannot be treated as they already have high levels of FSH, and any further attempted stimulation of the pituitary gland by administering FSH would be just like putting salt into the ocean.

Ovulation Induction with Tablets

In the presence of a normal or low FSH (there is little difference clinically whether the FSH is normal or low) the first line of treatment is usually oral tablets. In women with amenorrhoea, the first step is to bring on a menstrual bleed. Some doctors do a progestogen challenge test, where oral progestogen tablets are taken for 5–10 days, and the woman is then observed to see if she has a withdrawal bleed within a few days of withdrawing the progestogen. If she does (a positive test), that means she is likely to respond to OI tablets as there is some oestrogen secretion and some endometrium has been laid down, which then comes away when the progestogen level drops. The other option is to bring on a withdrawal bleed by administering the oral contraceptive pill (which contains both oestrogen and progestogen) for two to three weeks, and then await a withdrawal bleed. Even women with no oestrogen secretion should respond as the oestrogen component of the pill will stimulate some growth of the endometrium, which will come away when the hormones are stopped. After withdrawal bleeds, the first day of bleeding is counted as day one of the OI cycle. In women with spontaneous bleeding, the first day of a period can be taken as day one.

Several oral medications (often referred to as fertility pills) can be used, and the one that has been used the longest (for more than 50 years) is called clomiphene citrate. It is administered for five days early in the cycle (some doctors start day two, others day five) and the response can be monitored in several ways. Ultrasound examination (preferably through the vagina) can be used to watch the follicle(s) grow, and, all going well, then disappear as ovulation takes place, with the characteristics of the corpus luteum (described as a 'ring of fire') then being visible. By examining the ovary before ovulation, the number of growing follicles can be determined, and, if too many (more than three) are preovulatory in size (greater than 14 mm in diameter), it should be advised to avoid intercourse in that cycle because of the risk of multiple pregnancy.

However, using repeated ultrasounds is time consuming and expensive, but it is recommended that at least the first cycle should be monitored by at least one scan at about day 10–12 to exclude multiple follicular development. The most practical and most common method of monitoring ovarian response is to measure oestrogen and progesterone levels about three weeks into the cycle. A rise in oestrogen signifies that follicle(s) were growing, and a rise in progesterone signifies that ovulation has taken place. With this information, the plan for the next cycle can be made.

If there is little rise in oestrogen and no progesterone rise, it is clear that more stimulation and a higher dose of clomiphene citrate is required, increasing by a tablet for each daily dose (the usual starting dose is 50 mg per day and this should be increased to 100 mg). This can be repeated in the next cycles, up to a maximum of 200 mg per day. If there is still no response, OI using FSH injections should be considered (see later in the chapter).

If there is a good rise in oestrogen (suggesting follicular development) but no rise in progesterone, this suggests that follicle(s) grew but did not ovulate, and the positive feedback did not trigger an LH rise. In the next cycle, using the same dose of clomiphene citrate, an ultrasound can be performed at about day 12 looking for growing follicle(s). If there are not too many (three or fewer), ovulation is facilitated when the leading follicle is estimated to be preovulatory at about 16–18 mm in diameter. This is calculated by assuming that the leading follicle grows about 2 mm per day. Ovulation is triggered by administering HCG, a hormone that is chemically very similar to LH.

If there is ovulation as indicated by a rise in progesterone, the best-case scenario is that no period follows, and the woman has conceived.

In such a case, the OI is completed and we progress to pregnancy diagnosis. This is performed a few days after the due period and can be verified simply by a urine test done at home. A positive test is due to a rise in HCG hormone, which is secreted by the early embryo and enters the bloodstream, then excreted in the urine. Often in pregnancies achieved using OI, a more detailed pregnancy test is performed by actually measuring the blood concentration of HCG. Normal ranges of HCG have been determined for each stage of gestation in the first eight weeks of pregnancy.

An ultrasound at 6–7 weeks of estimated gestation is also recommended to confirm viability (that the pregnancy is progressing normally) and also to ensure that the pregnancy is a singleton rather than multiple (if more than one oocyte was ovulated and fertilised). Multiple pregnancy is a risk and is a recognised complication of OI, although with skilled use of clomiphene citrate, it should occur in fewer than 5% of pregnancies.

An often-confusing factor is when doctors talk about a 'six-week pregnancy' four weeks after the oocyte was fertilised. This is because in a conceptual cycle (where there is a pregnancy), the only known date with any certainty is the first day of the cycle, and that is also when the oocyte that became an embryo when fertilised started to grow. As such, when an embryo is formed about 14 days into the cycle, the pregnancy is already considered two weeks along its way. Using this system of dating, the average pregnancy is 40 weeks (280 days, or nine months plus seven days) in duration. Of course, not all babies are born on their due date, but most are born within 10 days of the due date (expected date of confinement [EDC]).

If ovulation has occurred, but there is no conception, then the same dose of clomiphene citrate should be prescribed again. We know from Chapter 1 that, apart from ovulation, the right number of fertile sperm must be placed in the right place at the correct time, so it is important that the male partner has a normal semen analysis. This should always be checked before OI. Furthermore, the woman's passages must be open and normal. If there is an obvious ovulation problem, and the woman has no risk factors for tubal damage (see Chapter 4), it is reasonable to proceed with OI on the basis that anovulation is the likely causative factor for the couple's failure to achieve a pregnancy. However, if no pregnancy is achieved after three ovulations, associated with well-timed intercourse with a fertile partner, then it is mandatory to check pelvic normality (See Chapter 4).

Other Oral Medications

Tamoxifen is used in a similar fashion to clomiphene citrate: at the beginning of the menstrual cycle for five days, at a dose of between 20 and 80 mg, dependent on response. Results obtained are similar to clomiphene citrate.

Letrozole is similar to clomiphene citrate, and pregnancy and complication rates are similar. It is now recommended by the 'International evidence-based guideline for the assessment and management of polycystic ovary syndrome 2018' as the first oral tablet to try in women who need OI and have PCOS.

About 80–90% of susceptible women will ovulate on oral treatment, but pregnancy rates are lower at about 60%. Keeping in mind that a fertile couple, on average, may take six months to conceive, several ovulations may be needed before conception. In addition to using ultrasound and hormone monitoring, it has always been the author's practice to suggest that women on OI with oral tablets also monitor their temperature chart. Not only will this give an indication of ovulation but it will also indicate when this occurred. The author also recommends that they have regular intercourse, and it is then possible to retrospectively check if timing was appropriate.

OI Using FSH Injections

The principle behind the oral OI agents is that they block the oestrogen receptors in the hypothalamic-pituitary-ovarian axis, which mitigates the negative feedback on FSH and results in elevated levels, which then stimulate the ovaries to produce mature follicles. This process is dependent on the hypothalamic-pituitary-ovarian axis being able to function normally.

In situations where this is not the case, they must be bypassed, whereas the ovary has to be stimulated directly. This is achieved by administering FSH hormone directly by injection, usually into the abdominal fat. Whereas with oral OI there is still a degree of negative feedback, and multiple pregnancies are infrequent, with FSH there is direct stimulation of the ovaries, and the opportunity for negative feedback is absent. Therefore, more rigorous monitoring is essential, and, even with utmost care, including ultrasound monitoring of follicular growth, the multiple pregnancy rate of successful treatment is about 20%. The rigorous monitoring may involve regular blood test for oestrogen levels and/or regular ultrasound monitoring of follicular growth (how many and how big). When the developing leading follicle(s) are estimated to reach preovulatory size, ovulation is triggered by administering HCG by injection. It is usual to check the hormone levels after ovulation, and often supporting smaller doses of HCG are administered every few days.

The commonest complication of FSH OI is the occurrence of multiple pregnancy. About one in five pregnancies are twins, with the occasional triplets. There is also a possibility of ovarian hyperstimulation syndrome (OHSS), with painful enlarged ovaries and fluid in the abdominal cavity (ascites). This is rare with OI and is far more common with stimulation for IVF. This will be discussed in Chapter 6. Because of the expense and complexity of FSH OI, it is good practice to confirm that the Fallopian tube(s) are open and that there is no other problem within the pelvis before starting treatment.

Polycystic Ovary Syndrome

One of the commonest causes of irregular, or failure of, ovulation is a condition called PCOS. It is now recognised that about one in five women, when examined by ultrasound, have polycystic ovaries (PCOs). These are seen on an ultrasound examination and show multiple small 'cysts' (less than 9 mm in

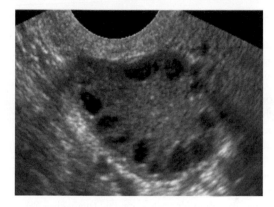

Figure 3.5   Ultrasound picture of a PCO showing about a dozen follicles around the periphery of the ovary in this one plane.

diameter) around the surface of one or both ovaries (see Figure 3.5). These 'cysts' represent follicles that have not matured but have come to the surface and have the potential to mature.

About half of the women who have PCOs have no symptoms, but, in the other half, there is a hormone imbalance of excess male hormone (androgen) secretion (these are testosterone and its metabolites: hormones derived from testosterone). This is accompanied by an excess secretion of LH. Symptoms may include obesity, excess hair growth (especially on the arms, legs and abdomen) and irregular periods or amenorrhoea. The condition was first described in 1935 by doctors Stein and Leventhal, and the syndrome was named after them. Today, it is known as PCOS.

The principles of OI in women with PCOS is similar to that described earlier in this chapter. However, as many of these women are overweight, the first line of treatment is diet and exercise. It is recognised that even a 5% loss of weight may restore spontaneous ovulation. Failing that, the next line of treatment is oral OI. Because of the many small follicles in the ovary, women with PCOS can be very responsive to stimulation, and a low dose is often used as a starting dose. Clomiphene citrate was the hormone that has been used since about 1961, but more recently it is recommended that letrozole (as described in the section 'Other Oral Medications' in this chapter) should be considered as the first line of pharmacological treatment. If oral tablets fail, then the next option is to use FSH OI. Again, such women may respond quickly, and occasionally can also get OHSS, so starting with a low dose and carefully monitoring by oestrogen hormone measurements and/or ultrasound scanning of the ovaries are required.

There is also a surgical option for treating anovulation in women with PCOS. When Stein and Leventhal first described the syndrome in 1935, they successfully treated it by operating on the ovary and removing a wedged section (bilateral wedge resection of the ovaries). When the oral OI agents became available, this treatment became obsolete. However, in the 1990s, when minimally invasive surgery/keyhole surgery became popular, there was a resurgence in an operative approach using laparoscopy (see Chapter 4) by a small telescope inserted into the abdominopelvic cavity. This technique is called laparoscopic ovarian drilling (LOD) and is performed using electric diathermy, laser generated heat or by simply pricking the cysts.

Although the mechanism of action of LOD is not understood, it does work. It has similar ovulation rates to FSH OI, does not cause multiple pregnancies nor does it require careful monitoring as it acts by restoring spontaneous natural ovulation. Its downside is that it requires a surgical procedure with its associated risks.

Summary

In conclusion, it can be said that virtually any woman who does not have ovarian failure with elevated FSH (absence of ovaries: born without or surgically removed, has not gone through the menopause, either naturally or prematurely) can be made to ovulate with appropriate treatment. However, even if a woman ovulates, there is no guarantee of pregnancy. First it must be highlighted again that it may take several ovulations. Second, ovulation is only part of the requirement for conception, and there is the need for the sperm and a normally functioning reproductive system (tubes, uterus and cervix). This is described in the following chapters.

4 Are My Uterus or My Tubes Stopping Me Getting Pregnant?

Chapter 1 explained that one of the three requirements for conception to happen is that the passages, the womb (uterus) and tubes (Fallopian tubes) have to be open and normal to allow the passage of sperm up, sweep the ovulated egg from the ovary into the funnel-like end of the Fallopian tube (the ampulla) and then transport the resulting embryo (after fertilisation) down the tubes into the uterus, where the embryo implants to establish a pregnancy (see Figure 4.1). As part of fertility investigations, it is important to exclude tubal damage, although tubal function cannot be assessed and must be implied from appearances. If the tubes are totally blocked, then this would explain the infertility. When the tubes are open but damaged, it is not possible to assess the chance of conception.

History

There is little in a woman's clinical history that can help with the diagnosis of fertility problems. Women who have had a sexually transmitted infection (STI), especially gonorrhoea or chlamydia, do have a risk of tubal damage, especially if there was more than one infection. Appendicitis is another significant risk factor, especially if the appendix had burst as the appendix is close to the right Fallopian tube and ovary.

Previous surgery in the pelvis is also a risk factor because of the possibility of postoperative pelvic adhesions, which may affect the tubes. Endometriosis can be difficult to diagnose on symptoms but can also be associated with pelvic infertility. The symptoms most likely to suggest endometriosis are

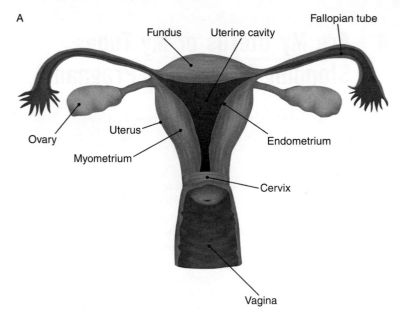

Figure 4.1 A. The female passages, uterus and Fallopian tubes. B. The female reproductive system.

painful periods, especially if the pain gets worse as menstruation progresses, and spotting before the period is established.

Examination

Doing a clinical examination will provide very little information about the status of the pelvis. Occasionally, enlargement of the uterus may suggest the presence of fibroids. Tenderness or thickening on either side of the uterus may indicate tubal inflammation. Ovarian cysts may be palpated (felt), or nodules suggesting the presence of endometriosis may be detected behind the uterus (Pouch of Douglas).

B

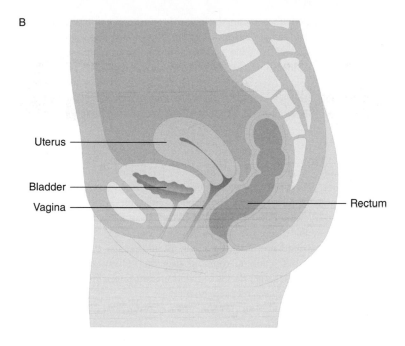

Figure 4.1 *(cont.)* SIDE VIEW

Imaging

X-ray

The early method of investigating tubal patency (i.e. whether the tubes are open) was to use X-ray technology, while injecting a radio-opaque (i.e. visible on X-ray examination) fluid through the cervix to outline the uterine cavity and the tubal channels (lumen), which shows up on the X-ray machine, and photographs on film can also be taken. This is called a hysterosalpingogram (HSG). While this test is helpful in diagnosing when the tubes are totally blocked, or if they are distended, it gives no information on the extent or severity of damaged tubes. It can also give false positives (when the tubes are not actually blocked but are in spasm), and it gives no information on the rest of the pelvis. However, it has the advantage that it can be performed by most radiology (X-ray) clinics and it does not require hospital admission nor anaesthesia, and it is often used as a screening test. Many women find it quite uncomfortable, and some find it painful. Some clinics still use HSG as a screening test, while others believe it has been superseded by other methods.

Ultrasound

While a basic ultrasonic examination of the pelvis is not helpful in confirming tubal patency, a modification of tubal imaging is to use ultrasound to visualise the pelvic organs while injecting some special fluid through the tubes, which can be seen with ultrasound: hysterosalpingo contrast sonography (HyCoSy). HyCoSy has similar diagnostic accuracy to an HSG. It has the benefit that it does not require X-radiation, is less painful, usually causing mild-to-moderate discomfort, and, while scanning, more information can be obtained about the ovaries and the uterus. Larger deposits of endometriosis (see the Endometriosis section later in this chapter) may also be seen.

Laparoscopy and Hysteroscopy

The 'gold standard' for investigating pelvic anatomy is the technique of laparoscopy. It was introduced to gynaecology in the English-speaking world in the 1960s by Dr Patrick Steptoe; better known for his role in producing the world's first test tube baby, Louise Brown (See Chapter 6). However, it requires surgery, usually on a day-surgery basis, and a general anaesthetic. After the patient is anaesthetised, a small needle is inserted under the belly button, and carbon dioxide gas is injected to distend the abdominal cavity. This elevates the abdominal wall from the bowel and pelvic organs, allowing the insertion of a trocar (a probe with a sharp point) and cannula, and, by replacing the trocar with the insertion of a telescope with a video camera attached to it (the laparoscope), the organs can be inspected (see Figure 4.2).

The laparoscope is then used to visualise the pelvic contents on a television screen to inspect the ovaries, the Fallopian tubes, uterus, appendix and the front of the rectum as well as the lining of the pelvis. Figure 4.3A shows a

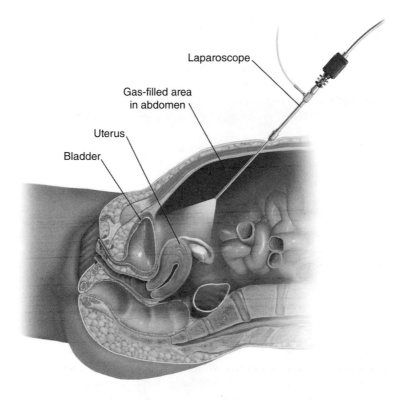

Figure 4.2 Laparoscopy: schematic drawing. The laparoscope is used for inspecting the pelvis and for keyhole surgery.

normal uterus and tubes. Other organs including the liver, bowel and gall bladder can also be inspected. To move the organs for better visualisation, a second probe is usually inserted at the pubic hairline. To assess whether the Fallopian tubes are open, saline coloured by methylene blue dye is injected through the vagina into the cervix and the uterine cavity, and its passage through the tubes is observed. The surgeon can see if the dye enters the tubes, how rapidly it flows and whether there is any obstruction, distension or complete blockage. With direct observation, any distension or irregularity of the tubes can be seen. It is also possible to inspect the finger-like protrusions

A

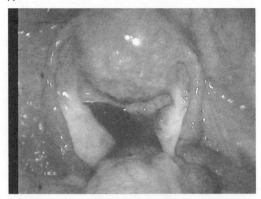

B

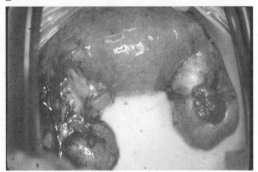

Figure 4.3   A. Laparoscopic picture of normal pelvis showing uterus, normal tubes and ovaries (white). B. Laparoscopy showing severe tubal adhesions and blockage.

(fimbriae) at the open end of the tubes as blunting or scarring suggests damage from inflammation. Sometimes the tubes can be completely blocked due to scarring, with total loss of fimbriae (Figure 4.3B).

Occasionally, scar tissue from previous infections can result in adhesions, and these act like cling film wrapping the ovaries, preventing the oocytes from entering the tubes. Adhesions around the tubes may prevent the fimbriae from reaching the ovarian surface to sweep the oocyte into the tubes. The ovaries

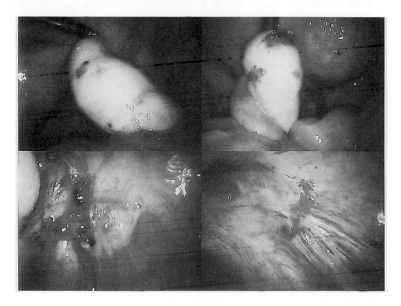

Figure 4.4 Endometriotic deposits on ovaries and endometriotic scarring in pelvis.

are also inspected, and signs of recent ovulation may be seen. The surgeon also surveys the whole pelvis, and looks for scar tissue from previous infections and for the presence of 'blood cysts', which indicate the presence of endometriosis (see Figure 4.4).

Laparoscopic examination is usually combined with inspection of the uterine cavity, again using a narrow telescope (called a hysteroscope) with a camera attached and a television screen. To enable inspection of the whole uterine wall, fluid is used to distend the cavity and it is examined for abnormalities such as scarring, polyps or fibroids (see Figure 4.5).

It is also usual practice to scrape the lining of the uterus (endometrium) for pathological examination. This will confirm if the endometrium is responding to the hormones appropriately and can confirm ovulation. It can also detect infections, such as tuberculosis, which still occurs in some countries. If abnormalities are detected, it is often possible to resect (surgically remove) scars, polyps and some fibroids using a broader operating hysteroscope. This

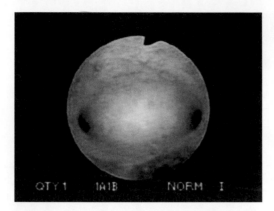

Figure 4.5 Hysteroscopic view of uterine cavity.

instrument has a double-channel cannula, with the telescope passing down one channel, and operating instruments such as scissors or forceps down the second. The commonest instrument used is called a wire loop, through which pulses of an electric current are passed, which heat the loop and enables it to cut away tissue, at the same time cauterising the underlying tissue, thereby minimising bleeding.

This technique is used for dividing scar tissue, removing polyps and resecting fibroids that protrude into the uterine cavity, all of which may prevent implantation. Sometimes a catheter that transmits laser energy is used instead of cautery. The small incisions used for a diagnostic laparoscopy are then closed with stitches, or sticking plaster, and the patient usually goes home the same day.

After effects of a diagnostic laparoscopy are usually mild. There may be some discomfort, often in the shoulders, which is caused by the carbon dioxide used during the procedure to distend the abdomen and allow the insertion of the trocar and cannulas and to allow space for operative procedures. There may also be some mild local pain from the incisions. Most women resume normal activity one to three days after the laparoscopy.

During the last 30 years, the practice of keyhole endoscopic surgery has developed. This enables surgery within the abdominal and pelvic cavities using the laparoscope with extra instruments being inserted through probes in the abdomen, which can include scissors and forceps, and even allows suturing (stitches) to be undertaken. Consequently, if there is scar tissue deforming or obstructing the tubes or covering the ovaries and inhibiting oocyte transport into the end of the Fallopian tubes, or deposits of endometriosis, these can be resected. Ovarian cysts can also be removed using the laparoscopic technique: this is called minimally invasive surgery.

Chapter 1 explained that the tubes are more than a piece of plumbing and that they have an intricate function. This requires not only that the tubes are open, but they are also able to fulfil their purpose. The cells lining the tubes need to be normal, and the hairs lining those cells (cilia), which are responsible for sweeping the gametes and embryo, need to be intact (see Figure 4.6).

Ultrasound and X-ray technology allows imaging of the tubal lumen, and laparoscopy enables looking at the tubes from the outside. However, as the

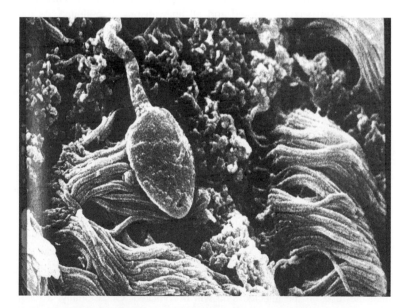

Figure 4.6 High-powered microscopy: a sperm in the Fallopian tube, showing the intricate structure of tubal lining with multiple folds and fine hairs (cilia).

tube has an intricate structure and has the important functions of transport and nutrition of the early embryo, it is useful to know what the lining looks like. An instrument called the falloposcope, which is a very thin telescope (0.5 mm in diameter), was developed in the 1990s, and can be passed into the tubal lumen through the uterine cavity using a hysteroscope, thus enabling inspection of the tubal lining. Unfortunately, the resolution of the falloposcope was inadequate to properly assess the lining, and the technique of falloposcopy has been abandoned.

The commonest cause of tubal damage is previous infection with inflammation, called salpingitis. This can be caused by pregnancy complications (miscarriage, abortion or after delivery if a small piece of the placenta is left behind and gets infected) from STIs, most often from chlamydia or gonorrhoea), and appendicitis or other infections in the abdominal cavity. STIs in women, in contrast to men who usually get significant pain on passing urine, often cause no symptoms and silently damage the tubes. In severe infections, the tubes can become blocked and fill up with pus (pyosalpinx). As the infection resolves, the pus changes to fluid (a fluid-filled tube due to infection is called a hydrosalpinx). Women with both tubes damaged and blocked cannot conceive as there is no passage between the oocyte and the sperm.

A common cause of tubal damage is after a tubal ectopic pregnancy. This occurs when the developing embryo implants but not within the uterine cavity. Most commonly, this is within the tubes, but it can also occur on the ovary and, rarely, on other pelvic organs. With a tubal ectopic pregnancy, there is usually pain and bleeding, and the diagnosis is made on ultrasound. Although these tubal pregnancies occasionally resolve without treatment (tubal abortion), they usually need medical or surgical treatment. If diagnosed early and there is minimal bleeding, administering a weak chemotherapeutic immunosuppressant (called methotrexate) can stop further development and solve the problem. Frequently, laparoscopic surgery is performed and, in the best-case scenario, the tube can be surgically opened, and the early products of conception sucked out. This preserves the tube, although some doctors believe that this will predispose to repeat tubal pregnancies. A more aggressive approach is to remove part or all the affected tube, which means that the tube on the affected side will be blocked. Occasionally, a tubal ectopic pregnancy will rupture and cause heavy bleeding into the peritoneal cavity (the internal contents of the abdomen and pelvis), presenting as a life-threatening emergency. This may require an incision into the abdomen and removal of the affected tube, again resulting in blockage.

Some believe that the cause of the ectopic pregnancy was previous tubal damage due to salpingitis, and, as this is usually bilateral (affecting both tubes), having had one tubal pregnancy predisposes to recurrence on the other side.

Open but Malfunctioning Tubes

As explained earlier in the beginning of this chapter, the tubes not only have to be open but also have to function normally with gamete/embryo transport and nutrition at a time when the embryo is growing from a single-cell zygote to a 100-cell blastocyst. The tubal lining is covered with cilia (as shown in Figure 4.6), which are important in the tube's transport role, and, if the cilia are damaged, the tube may not be able to function normally. With the disappointment that the falloposcope was not useful, there is no way of assessing the tubal lining as neither imaging nor laparoscopy can do this. Inspection of the finger-like ends of the Fallopian tubes can give some indication of the health of the tubes as these are the first to be damaged by infection; rather than acting like fingers sweeping the ovulated oocyte into the tubes, they act more like short thumbs, and so are less efficient. Thus, despite the tubes being open, they may be malfunctioning. There are other problems in the pelvis that can prevent conception, despite the tubes being open. Scar tissue around the ovary, which acts like cling film, may interfere with ovulation or prevent the oocyte entering the ampulla. This scar tissue may sometimes pull the ends of the tubes away from the ovary, making it less likely that the oocyte can find the opening. Another pelvic disease that can stop conception despite open tubes is endometriosis (see the Endometriosis section later in this chapter).

A common abnormality of the passages, especially as women age, is the presence of non-cancerous growths on the uterus called fibroids. Fibroids consist of 'swirls' of a combination of muscle and fibrous tissue, and they are quite common, especially as women age. They can occur within the uterine wall, projecting outwards, or project into the uterine cavity (called submucous fibroids). There is some debate about the significance of these fibroids in preventing implantation, but the consensus is that those that project into the uterine cavity are definitely a barrier to conception as they would prevent an embryo from implanting, and they should therefore be removed.

Submucous fibroids are often excised using the operating hysteroscope as described earlier in this chapter. Whether fibroids within the uterine wall or projecting from its surface are barriers to conception is still being debated, but they are sometimes removed for other reasons such as they are causing pressure symptoms or pain. The operating laparoscope can be used for smaller fibroids, whereas larger fibroids require surgery with an incision into the abdominal wall.

There is also consensus that polyps within the uterine cavity are also an obstacle to implantation and should be removed. This is usually performed through a hysteroscope with polyp forceps or cautery loop. It is a simple procedure done as day surgery.

Surgery is also indicated if the tubes are obstructed and contain fluids (hydro-salpinx), in which case they should be removed before contemplating IVF. It is felt that the fluid in the tubes may be hostile to the embryo and prevent its implantation. There are several studies to show that removing these tubes prior to IVF will result in higher success rates. Should it not be possible to remove hydrosalpinges, an alternative is to clip the proximal end so that fluid cannot escape into the uterine cavity.

Endometriosis

Endometriosis can prevent conception, even in the presence of open and normal looking tubes (this is discussed in detail in Chapter 5 in the section 'Other Problems: Endometriosis'). However, sometimes endometriosis can be responsible for significant damage and cause tubal obstruction. This can be due to either an endometriotic lesion on the tubes or scar tissue (adhesions) blocking the tubes. In women with subfertility, a surgical approach is usually tried to rectify the problem.

Surgical Treatment

The possibility of surgery resolving tubal infertility depends on the extent, the site and nature of the damage. The best scenario is a localised total blockage such as that caused by a previous tubal sterilisation. In this situation, the damaged segment can be resected and the tubes rejoined using microsurgery with an operating microscope. The use of the operating microscope was developed by plastic and reconstructive surgeons who needed to join arteries, nerves, tendons and other tissues with magnification. The technique was then introduced to gynaecology and tubal surgery, enabling surgery with magnification. This gives good results (at least 50% success) if there is only localised tubal damage, such as if clips were used for the previous tubal sterilisation. However, there is no surgery that can repair badly damaged tubal lining. Good results for tubal surgery are also achieved if the tubes are relatively normal but are caught up in external scarring (adhesions). Again, using either an operating laparoscope and keyhole surgery, or by opening the abdominal cavity (laparotomy) and using an operating microscope, these adhesions can be resected and tubal function may be restored.

A possible consequence of tubal surgery is that, if the damaged tube becomes open, fertilisation may take place, but there is a chance of the embryo getting stuck in the tube and resulting in a tubal ectopic pregnancy.

Other Solutions

Other solutions that have been tried but abandoned are tubal transplantation from a live donor and implantation of artificial tubes. Tubal transplantation required finding a tissue compatible donor and needed ongoing long-term immunosuppression. This was performed once between identical (monozygotic) twin sisters but was not successful. There was also no success in developing artificial tubes that could fulfil all the requirements.

Fortunately, IVF was developed in the 1970s, and today it is the most effective treatment for tubal infertility. This is discussed in detail in Chapter 6.

Myths

Again, we need to dispel a number of myths.

One myth is that, if the Fallopian tubes are blocked, they can easily be surgically unblocked. However, as has explained in this chapter, the tubes are not just pieces of plumbing joining the uterus to the ovary; they have an intricate function. Thus, there is more to tubal function than just 'open tubes'.

Another myth is that endometriosis can make a woman sterile. This is incorrect: women with extensive endometriosis can still conceive, as long as one of their tubes is patent.

5 Unexplained (Idiopathic) Infertility

Definition

Chapter 1 explained that the basic fertility factors were the right number of sperm, in the right place, at the right time, along with release of oocytes (eggs) and normal passages (the tubes and uterus). However, all these factors can appear adequate in some couples, yet no pregnancy results. These couples are said to have 'unexplained subfertility', the medical term being 'idiopathic subfertility'.

Causes

There are three possible reasons that could explain why no pregnancy has conceived. The first reason is a *transport problem*. This can happen when the oocytes are not captured by the finger-like projections (fimbriae) and so are not swept into the tubes, or not subsequently transported down the tube. Another transport problem is sperm not being able to get through the neck of the womb (cervix), the uterine cavity or the tubes. Transport problems also arise in the case of an early embryo down the tube; that is, an ectopic pregnancy.

The second reason is that of *failed fertilisation*. This happens in the outer third of the fallopian tube (ampulla), but there is no way of determining this.

The third possible reason is that of *implantation failure*. When the embryo arrives in the uterine cavity, it is made up of about 100 cells and is at the blastocyst stage (see Figure 1.4 in Chapter 1). It must then establish its root system and a circulation, which will eventually form the afterbirth (placenta). Even in the IVF process, failure of implantation is the biggest barrier, as it is in nature.

Transport

For many years, it was believed that the cervix with its mucus secretions was a possible barrier to sperm travelling towards the oocyte. We know that the mucus changes during the menstrual cycle, with the stretchy, clear, fertile mucus occurring just prior to ovulation. Is it possible that changes in the mucus at that time may prevent the sperm from penetrating it? As early as the 1860s, Dr J Marion Sims described the postcoital test (PCT), also called the Sims-Huhner test. He would instruct a couple to have intercourse before they came to consult him, and he would then suck out the cervical mucus, study it under the microscope, and, if he observed moving sperm, he came to three conclusions: First, the male was 'not barren'. Second, the 'cervix was in the right position to catch the sperm'. Third, if the sperm were moving, then 'the secretions were not inimical (hostile) to the sperm'. This test is not often used in the twenty-first century, and the author and colleagues' study in 1976 showed that more than half the women who came along for tubal sterilisation because they had as many children as they desired would fail a PCT. Consequently, the test was meaningless. It is also not a substitute for a semen analysis as it gives no indication of concentration, the quality of motility nor morphology.

We now understand that sperm can easily find their way to the cervix whatever its position, and that pregnancy can even occur occasionally with semen ejaculated on the vulva. Whether the cervix can be hostile to sperm is still debated. Some women do produce antisperm antibodies, which can be present in the blood and cervical mucus, but their significance is uncertain. Antibodies are produced by the white blood cells as part of the body's defence against infections or other foreign material. As sperm are a foreign material to a female, antisperm antibodies are produced in some women. These circulate in the blood and enter the cervical mucus, where they may impede the progress of these sperm on their way to the Fallopian tubes. However, antisperm antibodies can also be found in pregnant women, so they are not a complete block against sperm transport and do not always prevent conception.

Even if they are the suspected cause of a couple's failure to conceive, there is no proven specific treatment except IVF (see section 'The Role of IVF in Unexplained Subfertility' later in this chapter). Simply injecting the sperm through the cervix (AIH) will not solve the problem as the antibodies circulate in the blood and can have an effect in the uterus or tubes as well.

Artificial Insemination

Artificial insemination with a husband's or partner's semen is known as AIH or as intrauterine insemination. Doctors who believe that the cervix acts as a barrier will sometime suggest carrying out artificial insemination by injecting the partner's semen with a fine catheter through the cervix into the uterine cavity. This method has also been suggested when the male partner has suboptimal sperm, combined with a sperm-separation technique, where the best subsample of sperm is selected. The results are variable both as a treatment of male subfertility and for unexplained subfertility. Better success rates have been reported where the AIH process is combined with ovulation stimulation. Only low doses of FSH hormone are administered to try and avoid multiple pregnancies. Although some studies report improved pregnancy rates, up to one in three of these pregnancies are multiple, with their inherent complications. Pregnancy rates of 10% to 20% per cycle have been reported.

Fertilisation and Normal Development

There is no way of assessing fertilisation rate in the body as it can only be assessed if a couple undertakes IVF. With IVF, the number of oocytes inseminated or injected with sperm is known, and, the next day, the percentage that fertilise can be ascertained. If the rate is low (e.g. less than 30%), this would be considered as poor fertilisation rate and could be a reason for the subfertility. For a healthy baby to be born, the embryo must be normal with respect to its chromosome numbers; that is, euploid with 22 pairs of chromosomes plus two X or one X plus one Y chromosome. Again, in nature, this cannot be determined, but by combining genetic testing (see Chapter 6) and IVF, the embryo can be screened.

The Role of IVF in Unexplained Subfertility

When IVF is utilised as a treatment for unexplained subfertility, the first of the possible causes – transport – is eliminated as the sperm are placed together with the oocyte(s) in the laboratory. The day after the insemination, they are examined and the percentage that are fertilised is assessed. The normal fertilisation rate is about 60%–70%. Should the fertilisation rate be significantly lower, fertilisation failure may be the reason for the subfertility. Should a pregnancy not occur with any available embryo(s), in subsequent cycles ICSI should be used (the indication being poor fertilisation rate) and it is likely to overcome this with a better fertilisation rate and more embryos available for transfer and freezing.

Implantation

The diagnosis of implantation failure is a diagnosis of exclusion; that is, the transfer of euploid normal-looking embryos have not resulted in pregnancy. The physiology of implantation was discussed in Chapter 1, and this is a complex process. Initially, the blastocyst must reach the receptive endometrium, there must be apposition, then attachment of the blastocyst, and finally invasion. Half of the embryo's material comes from the father, so this is foreign material as far as the immune system of the female is concerned. Yet, under the right circumstances, the embryo manages to invade the endometrium without being attacked and rejected by the immune system. This is due to the endometrium being considered an immunologically privileged site but the mechanism of how this has developed is not understood. The process of invasion and placentation is complex and involves many chemical enzymes and biochemical factors. While our understanding of these factors is improving, there is still no test that can be used to assess the ability of the endometrium to accept an embryo, nor can anything be done to enhance this.

The third possible cause of unexplained subfertility, implantation failure, cannot be diagnosed by IVF, but replacing the embryo through the cervix into an optimised endometrium may bypass the problem without making a diagnosis. Experience shows that success rates for couples undergoing IVF for unexplained subfertility are similar to those who are being treated for tubal or male-factor subfertility.

Other Problems: Endometriosis

A common finding in women with subfertility is endometriosis. This is a condition where some of the glandular lining of the womb grows outside the uterine cavity. This can be within the muscular wall of the uterus (myometrium), which is then called adenomyosis, or outside the womb: on the ovaries, pelvic wall, bowel, bladder, virtually anywhere in the pelvic cavity or the abdomen. How this endometrium gets outside the uterine cavity is not known. It may spill out along the tubes, flow through blood vessels or seed through the lymphatic system, or it may simply grow in an abnormal area. It is believed that women who get endometriosis may have a different immune system to other women, which fails to 'mop-up' the misplaced tissue.

The severity of the condition varies from one or two spots the size of a pinhead, to large ovarian cysts consisting of endometrial lining and containing old blood (which looks like chocolate), known as chocolate cysts. With severe endometriosis, the tubes can be covered in scar tissue (adhesions) and even be blocked, the ovaries can be distorted, or the endometriotic scars can cover the uterus, bowels and bladder, and even obstruct the flow from the kidneys to the bladder (ureters). Even if the endometriosis does not cause a mechanical barrier to egg/sperm/embryo transport, chemicals called prostaglandins are secreted, which can interfere with transport and implantation. The mechanism of how this happens is not really understood.

Symptoms depend on the site of deposits but are not necessarily affected by the severity of the condition. Mild deposits can cause severe pain, and large lesions my cause little or no pain. The commonest complaint is painful periods; pain that gets worse as menstrual flow progresses. Pain during intercourse can occur if there are deposits near the vagina, and pain on bowel movements if the bowel is involved. If there are adhesions, pain may be felt throughout the cycle. A warning sign may be menstrual spotting prior to full menstruation. If the disease is severe and it obstructs the tubes, this will obviously cause problems with conceiving. However, even minimal amounts of endometriosis may be associated with subfertility. It is believed that the endometriotic deposits secrete hormones called prostaglandins, which can interfere with all aspects of fertilisation and implantation.

The diagnosis of endometriosis can only be made by seeing the lesions at laparoscopy or at open operation on the pelvis, thus it often goes undiagnosed. A suspicion may be raised on a blood test for CA125, a biochemical marker that is often elevated in endometriosis, but there are other causes of an elevated level of CA125. Ovarian endometriotic cysts are usually seen on ultrasound, and scarring behind the uterus caused by endometriosis may also have a characteristic appearance on ultrasound. However, the gold standard is to see deposits on laparoscopy, with a biopsy taken for confirmation under the microscope by a pathologist.

Although subfertility is frequently associated with endometriosis, there are many women who do conceive, despite having the condition. Furthermore, if a woman with endometriosis conceives, the disease usually improves during pregnancy. Consequently, one of the common treatments is to use a progesterone-like hormone (a progestogen), which suppresses the growth of uterine lining inside and outside the uterus. Various progestogens have been used, taken by mouth, vaginally, rectally or by injection.

An alternative way of suppressing endometrium is to administer hormones that prevent the release of hormones from the pituitary (especially FSH) so that follicles do not develop in the ovary, and oestrogen hormone is not secreted or circulated in the blood. As the proliferation of the endometrium is dependent on oestrogen, this oestrogen-deficient state results in the endometrium dying off (atrophy).

A popular way of suppressing growth of endometrium was to administer an androgenic (male-type hormone) called danazol taken by mouth, which then stops menstruation and suppresses the endometriotic deposits. Unfortunately, it has significant masculinising side effects, such as fluid retention, acne, hair growth and even voice change. Some women found it greatly increased their sex drive (libido).

A similar effect of suppressing follicular development and a consequent oestrogen-deficient state could be achieved by administering a GnRH agonist (see Chapter 6). Although a daily injection is used for IVF, with pituitary suppression, a pellet can be implanted under the skin, which will secrete hormones and be effective for three months. An alternative route of administering GnRH is by daily nasal spray. GnRH is very effective in reducing circulating oestrogen to levels women experience in the menopause. Although this treatment is also effective in suppressing endometrial deposits, it is also associated with side effects similar to those in menopausal women: hot flushes and dry vagina during intercourse. There is also some concern that prolonged usage may accelerate thinning of the bones (osteoporosis), but the usual course of six months is probably not a significant risk.

Although minor lesions can be treated with hormones, the mainstay of treatment of endometriosis today is surgery. This can be minor surgery using laparoscopy with excision or destruction of lesions, using an electric current (diathermy), laser energy or laparoscopic scissors passed down an operating channel. Excision is now the preferred method. An operating robot is sometimes used, especially if the laparoscopic operation is a lengthy procedure.

Postoperatively, hormones are sometime administered as an adjunct to surgical treatment.

It is also recognised that women may conceive despite having a degree of endometriosis. Although there is some argument about whether mild degrees of endometriosis should be treated, the consensus is that, if endometriosis is associated with subfertility, and there is no other apparent cause, then the pelvis should be normalised before proceeding to other treatments. This also applies to women planning IVF.

There are many reports in the literature claiming postsurgery pregnancy rates of 30%–90%, but randomised controlled trials are difficult to undertake as each patient is so different.

The treatment of a woman with endometriosis must be discussed with her treating doctor. Even after successful treatment of endometriosis, it is possible for the lesions to return.

Much research still needs to be done on what causes this condition, whether it can be prevented and what the best treatments are. It is such an important condition, that the World Endometriosis Society (WES) has been established to promote such research. The WES advances evidence-based standards and innovations for education, advocacy, clinical care and research in endometriosis, adenomyosis and related disorders in collaboration with its stakeholders and global partners to improve the lives of all affected women and their families.

6 What Is IVF and What Does It Entail?

History

As described in Chapter 4, the tubes (Fallopian tubes) are intricate structures, which are easily damaged. Although tubal microsurgery was introduced into gynaecology in the 1970s, the results of operating on damaged tubes were disappointing. This is understandable because of their intricate structure. Even when blocked tubes were reopened (i.e. patency was restored), the tubes still sometimes did not work normally. Other strategies were therefore called for. With the developments in organ transplantation, attempts were made to transplant healthy Fallopian tubes from a donor who did not wish to have children to someone whose damaged tube would be removed and replaced by the normal tube. This, however, required lifelong immunosuppression to avoid rejection, and was not feasible, and the one reported attempt did not work. Another 'out-of-the-box' solution that was attempted was to cover the ovaries in a plastic envelope and drain these with artificial tubes into the uterine cavity. Again, and not surprisingly because of the intricate function of the Fallopian tubes, this attempt did not work. Consequently, another solution was needed.

A solution that seemed feasible was to remove oocytes from a woman, mix them with her partner's sperm in the laboratory and, after the oocyte was fertilised by sperm (IVF: in vitro fertilisation; meaning 'in-glass fertilisation'), grow the embryo in the test tube for a few days and then transfer it into the woman's uterus. This technique had already been applied in animals, initially in rabbits (first attempted in the 1930s) and later in mice, guinea pigs and even sheep. Its application to humans was first attempted by John Rock and Miriam

Menkin at Harvard Medical School in the USA in 1944. Although they successfully achieved IVF of a human oocyte, they did not attempt replacement of the embryo. There are no further reports on inseminating human eggs in vitro until 1965, with the publication in the prestigious medical journal, *The Lancet*, by Robert ('Bob') Edwards. He had great difficulty finding collaborators among British gynaecologists, and it was following his time spent at John Hopkins Medical School in Baltimore USA in collaboration with Howard and Georgeanna Jones that he reported on the maturation of human oocytes in vitro. After returning to Cambridge, he had a chance meeting with Patrick Steptoe in 1968, who was an expert in gynaecological laparoscopy, and they eventually teamed up at Kershaw's Cottage Hospital in Oldham, Manchester. Steptoe collected oocytes from women using the operating telescope, and then passed them to the laboratory of Bob Edwards, which they established near the operating room. In 1969, they reported on the fertilisation and cleavage in the laboratory of these human oocytes in another prestigious medical journal, *Nature*. The newspapers reported on their paper with sensational headlines such as: 'This human time bomb' and 'Next chance to choose baby's sex' (*Daily Mail*), 'Move towards test tube babies' (*Times of London*), 'Test tube baby factory' (*Sunday Mirror*) and 'Life outside the body' (*Daily Express*).

Edwards received criticism from his colleagues (who resented his attention from the press), and research funding from the Medical Research Council (MRC) was refused in 1971 on the basis that the research 'bristles with difficulties practical, ethical and financial'. Requests to have Patrick Steptoe appointed to the clinical school in Cambridge to save Bob Edwards travelling for over three hours each way were also refused. Consequently, Patrick Steptoe had to continue his egg collections in Oldham and Bob Edwards had to travel nearly 200 miles each way to work in the adjoining laboratory. In the 1960s and 1970s, the focus on reproductive research was on contraception to control the population explosion, and the general opinion was that infertility was not a problem worth investing in. Even more importantly, because infertility was not seen as a problem worth solving, or able to be solved by IVF, the women undergoing the procedures were seen as experimental subjects and not as patients undergoing experimental treatments. Even the Nobel laureate, James Watson (who co-described the double-helix DNA) suggested at a meeting in Washington DC, where Bob Edwards spoke, that IVF would 'produce monster babies'.

Then, in 1971, Professor Carl Wood's team in Melbourne also started working on human IVF and achieved a pregnancy in 1973, but unfortunately it was short-lived and only lasted for a few days: a biochemical pregnancy. Interestingly, a Ford Foundation grant, which the Melbourne team was awarded in 1976, was because the funders hoped that research into IVF might have spin-offs for fertility control. Furthermore, the Ford Foundation stated that, if the team achieved a success, the Foundation did not wish to be named. After 40 attempts at embryo transfer, Steptoe and Edwards achieved their first pregnancy in 1976, but this was another disappointment with the pregnancy growing in the Fallopian tube   an ectopic pregnancy – and it had to be surgically removed.

Steptoe and Edwards continued their attempts, and their one-hundred-and-second transfer resulted in the birth of Louise Brown, the world's first IVF baby born, who was on 25 July 1978. Although Bob Edwards had attempted to stimulate the ovary to make multiple oocytes using fertility hormones, none of those cycles were successful, and Louise Brown was born from a natural cycle with only one oocyte collected and inseminated, with the embryo transferred at the eight-cell stage. The first Australian baby, Candice Reed (third in the world) born in June 1980, was also conceived in a natural cycle. Meanwhile, Carl Wood's team in Melbourne persevered with using hormonal stimulation and showed that these stimulated cycles could work, having produced 10 babies in 9 women during 1981 (the world's fourth to thirteenth). Using stimulation, success rates of about 10% were obtained, which converted IVF from a rare success of an experimental procedure to a feasible option, albeit with limited success. Consequently, today IVF is almost always performed in stimulated cycles using COH.

The opposition to IVF did not end after Louise Brown was born in July 1978. The press was generally positive about the birth as a British success, and *The Times* complimented Edwards and Steptoe on perfecting the technique 'against enormous odds'. The MRC changed its attitude in 1978/79 and sanctioned IVF: 'Human IVF with subsequent embryo transfer should now be regarded as a therapeutic procedure covered by normal doctor/patient ethics'. The hostility was also experienced in Australia: the churches (both Catholic and Anglican) lobbied for IVF to be banned, feminists opposed IVF because they said it was 'male doctors experimenting on women' and the antiabortion 'Right to Life' groups objected on religious grounds.

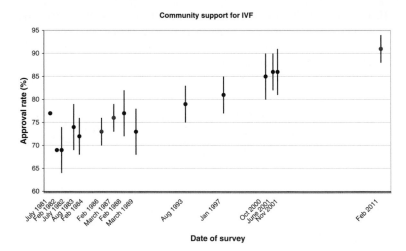

Figure 6.1   Response to community surveys with approval rates for IVF to help infertile couples, shown as percentage of respondents with standard error (where available).

When applied modifications such as embryo freezing were announced, many thought that the 'brave new world' had arrived and that IVF was progressing too quickly.

To assess what the community really thought, the author and colleagues carried out a number of community surveys by Morgan Gallop Polls, a respected market research group, over a 30-year period (1981–2011) (see Figure 6.1). This showed that the community's attitude to using IVF to help infertile couples have children has always had majority approval, rising from about 70% in 1981 to over 90% in 2011. Over the last four decades, opposition has waned but there are still some opponents of reproductive technology, especially when it applies to the more unusual forms of parenting such as egg, sperm or embryo donation and surrogacy.

Step One: Controlled Ovarian Hyperstimulation

The theory behind using stimulated cycles is that, if several oocytes can be collected, a batch of embryos may be produced and this would give the option to select the best embryo(s) for transfer. Because initial success rates were low, it was quite common to replace several embryos – often three – and sometimes more. This could result in a multiple pregnancy with its associated complications. Today – virtually always – a single embryo only is transferred. Fortunately, success rates with single-embryo transfers these days are higher than with the triple embryo transfers in the 1980s.

The initial attempts at stimulating the ovary involved using an oral-ovulation induction agent – clomiphene citrate – in a dose of 150 mg for five days. Soon, the regimen was changed to using FSH, which was purified from the urine of postmenopausal women. Such women have high blood levels of FSH (where the hypothalamic-pituitary-ovarian axis is attempting to stimulate the fading ovary), which is then excreted into the urine, collected and purified. By the turn of the century, FSH was produced purely in the laboratory by a molecular biology technique called recombinant DNA technology. This has the advantage that It Is synthetically produced, is available in unlimited supply and is consistent in concentration.

The aim is to prescribe a dose of FSH that will result in 15–20 maturing follicles in the two ovaries, which would hopefully result in 12–15 oocytes being collected for IVF. Several factors are taken into consideration when the starting dose of FSH for the first stimulated IVF cycle is prescribed. Most important is the number of follicles on a baseline scan undertaken in the month(s) before stimulation commences. This gives an indication of the number of potential follicles in the ovary that can respond to stimulation. The other important factor is the AMH concentration (see Chapter 2), which is measured before treatment starts. Response to any previous FSH administration is also relevant, as is a woman's FSH level in the blood, her age and her body weight. The FSH is administered by daily injection subcutaneously (into the fatty tissue) usually in the abdominal wall. This is administered for 10–14 days until sufficient follicles have developed to a size, which indicates that the oocyte within is mature. Although the dose can be adjusted during the stimulated cycle, it is the starting dose that determines how many follicles are recruited to form the cohort that started to grow at the start of the cycle.

Step Two: Monitoring

Follicular growth is monitored by examining the ovaries using ultrasound technology, through the vagina (see Figure 6.2). This enables the number of

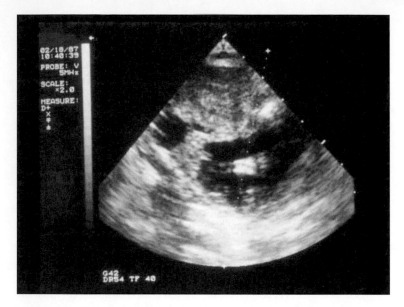

Figure 6.2 Ultrasonic scan of stimulated ovary. The 'black holes' represent stimulated follicles, with the dotted line showing where the aspiration needle will pass.

developing follicles and their size to be determined. Using ultrasound, when the oocyte within a follicle is mature and is ready to be collected, the follicular diameter is about 16–20 mm. Each clinician has their own regimen of follicular monitoring, but at least one ultrasound scan should be undertaken on about the eighth or ninth day of stimulation. As follicles grow at about 2 mm in diameter per day, it can be estimated when the oocytes may be ripe and ready for ovulation.

Some clinics also use hormone measurements, especially oestrogen, which has two benefits. First, a rising level of oestrogen confirms that the follicles are maturing, and second, a rapid rise or high level of oestrogen in the blood is a warning that too many follicles are developing and the woman may be at risk of OHSS (see below). In the early days of IVF when ovulation was spontaneous, women had to be carefully monitored for ovulation so that oocytes could be collected before the follicles ruptured, but now we are able to prevent spontaneous ovulation.

First, two types of hormones can be used to inhibit premature ovulation by inhibiting the release of the LH; these are GnRH agonists and GnRH antagonists. They both achieve the same outcome but by different means. The agonists act by strongly stimulating the pituitary gland and releasing all the gonadotrophins, and then inhibiting the production of any further of these hormones. The antagonists act by blocking the GnRH receptor in the pituitary immediately, thus preventing LH release. The result of both treatments is that LH hormone is not secreted, and, without the important LH peak, the follicles are not triggered to ovulate.

The second part of controlling the cycle is the ability to trigger follicles to bring the oocytes to maturity. The most common way to achieve this is by administering a dose of HCG, which has a biological action very similar to LH, and triggers final maturation of the oocyte, and subsequent ovulation 36–40 hours later. In a stimulated COH cycle, HCG is administered when the follicles are judged to contain almost mature oocytes and the oocyte collection is then performed 32–36 hours later, just before the expected ovulation. Just as recombinant FSH has replaced urinary FSH, recombinant HCG (rHCG) is now also available.

In an antagonist cycle, another option to trigger final maturation is to use a GnRH agonist trigger. Administering a dose of GnRH agonist to a woman who has been stimulated with FSH and using GnRH antagonist will result in a surge of natural LH from the pituitary gland, which then stimulates final oocyte maturation/ovulation. This protocol is always used if the woman is making too many oocytes and is at risk of OHSS, as this is less likely if HCG is not administered.

The hormones used in an IVF cycle are summarised in Table 6.1.

OHSS occurs when there is an excessive response to FSH and too many follicles are developing, releasing large amounts of oestrogen. OHSS causes the ovaries to swell and become painful. Women become bloated, and they may be nauseated, develop shortness of breath, have decreased urination and have excessive weight gain. There is also the risk of blood clots forming. Some women are ill enough to be admitted to hospital, sometimes even into intensive care units. OHSS usually resolves on its own within a week or two but may take somewhat longer if the woman conceives. Treatment is supportive, keeping the woman comfortable, and avoiding complications.

Medication	Indication
Clomiphene/clomifene	A tablet that stimulates ovarian follicles to grow
FSH Urinary FSH (uFSH) – purified from the urine of menopausal women	This hormone is the main one used to stimulate multiple follicular development
Recombinant FSH (rFSH) Produced in the laboratory	Both uFSH and rFSH have similar actions
GnRH agonist	A hormone that inhibits ovulation by depleting LH from the pituitary It can also be used to trigger ovulation in an 'antagonist' cycle
GnRH antagonist	A hormone that inhibits ovulation by blocking the release of LH from the pituitary
HCG	Used to trigger ovulation
Progesterone Vaginal pessary or intramuscular injection	Administered after oocyte collection to change the endometrium to secretory (receptive)

Table 6.1 Hormones used during an IVF cycle

Step Three: Oocyte Collection

Originally, the technique used for collection of oocytes was using the operating telescope (laparoscope) pioneered by Patrick Steptoe. In the mid-1980s, the use of ultrasound for oocyte collection was developed by Wifred Feichtinger in Vienna, initially through the abdominal wall, and later through the vagina. Today, the ultrasound-guided transvaginal oocyte collection is standard practice around the world.

Ultrasound-guided transvaginal oocyte collection can be performed in a procedure room with light sedation and local anaesthesia, or in an operating room with intravenous sedation or even general anaesthesia. The technique used depends on the clinic and the clinician.

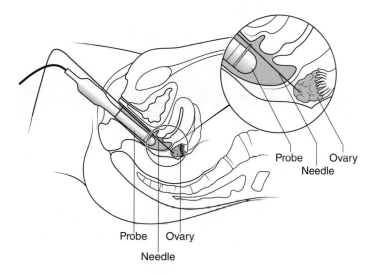

Probe | Ovary
Needle

Probe | Ovary
Needle

Figure 6.3 Ultrasound-guided oocyte collection. The ultrasound probe enables visualisation of the follicles within the ovaries (see Figure 6.2) and a guideline on the screen shows where the aspiration needle will pass.

Oocyte collection is performed by inserting the vaginal ultrasound probe and visualising the ovaries. The developed follicles can then be identified and, with a calibrated channel using ultrasound guidance, an aspiration needle is inserted into each follicle (see Figure 6.3) and its fluid is aspirated using a foot-operated suction pump, which is attached to the needle. It is not usually possible to see the oocytes with the naked eye, thus the follicular fluid is passed to an embryologist (a scientist who specialises in IVF) who inspects it under the microscope (see Figure 6.4A). When identified, the oocyte is removed with a pipette and placed in another dish containing a specially prepared solution (culture media) (see Figure 6.4B). It is then kept at body temperature in a special oven (incubator) until it is ready to be combined with sperm (insemination).

This is then repeated until all visible follicles of reasonable size have been drained. If there is difficulty in obtaining oocytes by simple aspiration, the follicles can be flushed with culture medium to try and flush out the oocyte.

A

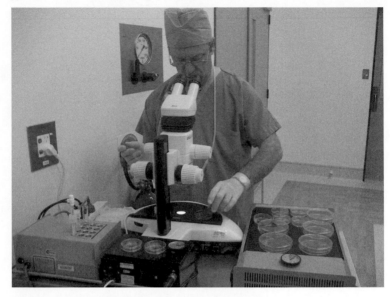

B

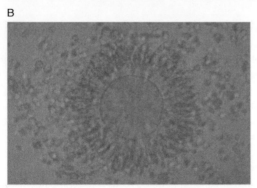

Figure 6.4   A. An embryologist inspecting follicular fluid under a microscope. B. Oocyte as seen under the microscope after collection.

A

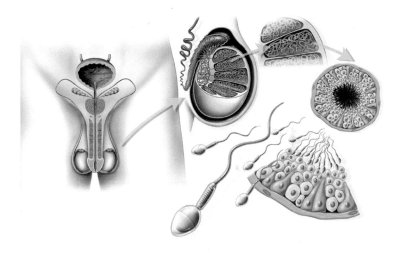

Figure 1.2 The male reproductive system. A. The testicle and its duct system. B. A single sperm as seen under the microscope.

B

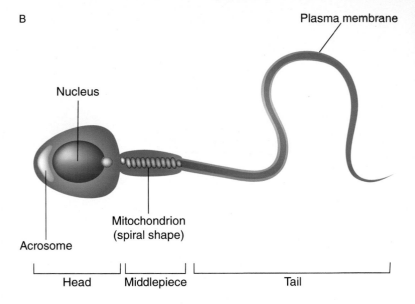

Figure 1.2 (*cont.*)

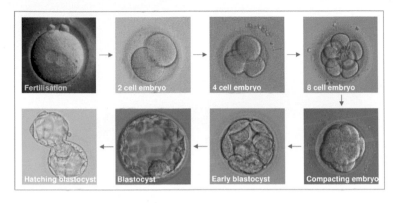

Figure 1.4 Embryo development from a fertilised oocyte to blastocyst stage.

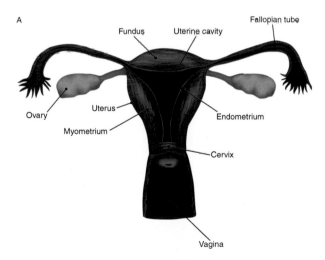

Figure 4.1 A. The female passages, uterus and Fallopian tubes. B. The female reproductive system.

B

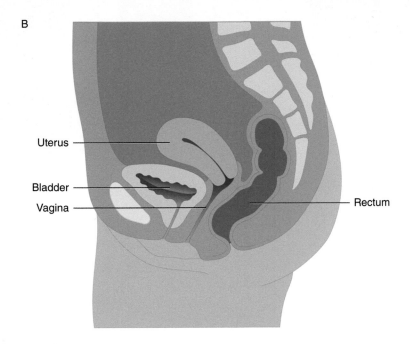

Uterus

Bladder

Vagina

Rectum

Figure 4.1 *(cont.)*

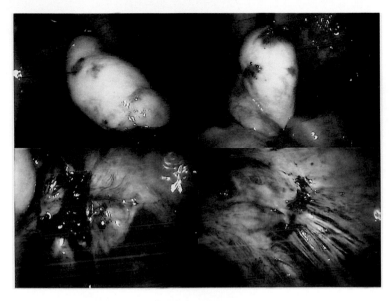

Figure 4.4 Endometriotic deposits on ovaries and endometriotic scarring in pelvis.

A

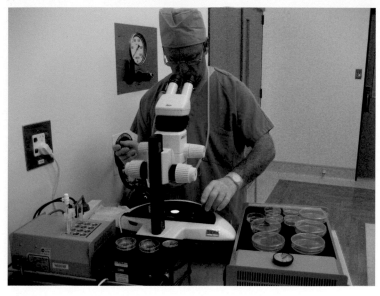

Figure 6.4 A. An embryologist inspecting follicular fluid under a microscope. B. Oocyte as seen under the microscope after collection.

Figure 6.4 (*cont.*)

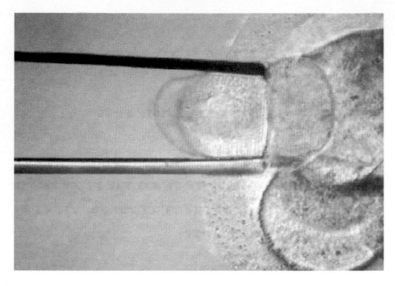

Figure 6.5 The removal of a single blastomere (cell) from an eight-cell embryo.

After completion of the procedure, the woman then rests in the recovery ward for an hour or two, and she is then discharged home.

Step Four: Laboratory Procedures of Fertilisation (With Possible ICSI) and Embryo Culture

While the oocytes are being collected, the male partner produces a semen sample by masturbating into a sterile jar. If he cannot be present at the time of the oocyte collection, it is possible for him to provide a sample in advance, which is then frozen, stored and defrosted after the oocytes have been collected. If the male does not have sperm in his ejaculate, surgical removal of sperm from the testicle or vas is undertaken, as described in Chapter 3. The sperm is kept at body temperature, mixed to a liquid consistency and prepared for insemination. In natural conception, the selection of the sperm that will fertilise the oocyte out of the 200 000 000 ejaculated is a very sophisticated process. Replicating this in the laboratory requires the isolation of the high-quality subsample of sperm and separating those sperm from the ejaculate, which also contains dead or immotile sperm, immature sperm, white blood cells, bacteria and other cellular debris.

Several techniques have been developed to try and extract the best sperm from the complex melange. The principal step is to flow the semen through a filter called gradient centrifugation, which selects sperm which are believed to be the ones most likely to achieve fertilisation. Sometimes chemicals are added to enhance motility, and sometimes the specimen is passed through a glass wool column. In standard IVF, there is a resemblance to nature in that the ovum selects which sperm will penetrate its outer shell (ZP), which acts as a filter to exclude any spermatozoa that it does not consider suitable.

If there are insufficient sperm present to achieve fertilisation by standard IVF, the microinjection technique of ICSI is used (see Figure 2.3 in Chapter 2). With this technique, only one sperm is required for each oocyte, and the selected sperm is injected into the substance (cytoplasm) of the oocyte. With ICSI, it is the embryologist who selects the sperm, so selecting normal-looking sperm is important. However, it is hard to tell if the sperm is normal just by inspecting it under the microscope; it is like assessing a used car by just looking at its body. To find the most normal sperm with the least DNA damage, tests to assess the degree of DNA damage are being developed (including tests called Comet, TUNEL, SCSA and SCD). However, studies utilising these tests have inconsistent findings, and it is not clear what role they have in selecting the best sample.

Once the oocytes have been inseminated or microinjected, they are placed in culture medium in an incubator, which is a type of oven that controls temperature, oxygen and carbon dioxide concentrations, and humidity. The oocytes are observed about 18 hours after insemination or injection for signs of fertilisation: the presence of two pro-nuclei (see Figure 1.4 in Chapter 1). Some incubators are now fitted with video cameras, which take many pictures of the developing embryo(s) during their culture. This is called time-lapse photography and its proponents believe it enables selection of the embryos that are more likely to result in pregnancy. If time lapse is not used (and its use is not routine in most clinics), the embryologist selects the best-looking embryo(s) for transfer and those suitable for freezing by morphological appearance, such as the speed of development of the embryo, the number of cells at each inspection and the uniformity of cell size.

The embryos are cultured for three to five days, followed either by daily inspection under the microscope or by studying the time lapse. Some time-lapse incubators use artificial intelligence to select the 'best' embryos by studying their development compared to millions of stored images of developing embryos that have resulted in normal births. There is now a simpler process without time lapse but using artificial intelligence, looking at still photos that also suggest which is the embryo most likely to result in an ongoing pregnancy. Evidence is still lacking to show that this method is more effective than selection by an experienced embryologist.

In the early days, several embryos were transferred to improve the chance of success. This, however, resulted in multiple pregnancies (twins, triplets, quadruplets, and so on). While such pregnancies were considered IVF successes, they were high risk with premature births and their complications. Consequently, the number of embryos transferred has been reduced, and most transfers today are only single-embryo transfers. Reassuringly, the chance of pregnancy with a single-embryo transfer today is much higher than it was with three embryos 30 years ago.

Step Five: Embryo Transfer

The final step in a 'fresh' IVF cycle is the transfer of the developing embryo from the culture medium in the incubator in the laboratory into the uterine cavity. This is called the embryo transfer (ET). It is the last step in the reproductive technology marathon, and pregnancy depends on its successful accomplishment. The process involves loading the embryo under the microscope into a fine catheter in a small volume of culture medium, then introducing the catheter through the cervix into uterine cavity and slowly injecting the small volume of fluid containing the embryo. The process is similar to having a smear test performed, which most women have experienced.

Initially it was done 'blindly', calculating the distance that the catheter was passed depending on the length of the uterine cavity from preoperative ultrasound measurement. Today, most clinics use ultrasound control by holding the ultrasound transducer on the abdomen and actually visualise the catheter being passed into the uterine cavity. The embryo is then slowly expelled within the drop of culture medium.

When the first pregnancies were achieved, women had to lie in bed for 24 hours with minimal movement after ET. With more experience, it was proven that this makes no difference as the embryo does not 'fall out'. Consequently, today the woman rests for a few minutes only, and then can resume activities. In the first three decades of IVF, embryos were transferred when the cells just commenced dividing – cleavage stage – two or three days after insemination/ICSI. With improved culture media and techniques including time-lapse incubators, the standard practice today is to grow embryos in vitro for five days, until they are made up of about 100 cells at the blastocyst stage (see Figure 1.4 in Chapter 1). This allows for a better selection of viable embryos that are likely to survive. Once the ET has been performed, the fresh cycle is completed. Usually, hormones are prescribed to boost the hormone level in the luteal phase. This is routinely used in cycles where a GnRH agonist was used.

If embryos are produced that are judged to be able to survive freezing and thawing, then these can undergo preservation, which is the sixth step in the IVF process: cryopreservation.

Step Six: Embryo Freezing

Should pregnancy not result with the fresh ET, the option of repeated attempt (s) using the frozen embryo(s) – if they are available – can be undertaken. If the fresh ET is successful, then the embryo(s) can be stored for years until required for subsequent pregnancies.

The technique of freezing embryos was developed in animal husbandry using liquid nitrogen with embryos being cooled slowly. It was necessary to cover the embryos in a solution to protect the cells during freezing and thawing, when ice crystals can form and damage the cells. The technique has now changed to vitrification (glass like), a technique whereby the embryos are frozen rapidly, going from room temperature to –196°C in less than a second, and this avoids crystal formation. This is a far more effective technique to freeze blastocysts than the early slow-freeze method used for cleavage-stage embryos and achieved survival rates of 70%–80%. Using vitrification and subsequent warming is associated with superior survival and pregnancy rates, so this is the method of choice today. The frozen embryos can then be warmed one at a time and replaced either in natural cycles – where the time of ovulation is monitored and they are replaced at the appropriate time corresponding to when they were frozen (usually day five or six) – or in cycles where hormones are used to stimulate the uterine lining, called hormone replacement therapy (HRT) cycles. In HRT cycles, hormones are administered usually as oestrogen tablets alone for 10–14 days to build up the endometrium, and its thickness can be checked using ultrasound. Then progesterone is added, usually as pessaries, to mimic the postovulation changes in the lining. The embryo is then replaced after five days of progesterone use if it was frozen on day five after insemination.

The six steps of an IVF cycle are summarised in Table 6.2.

Preimplantation Genetic Diagnosis and Embryo Biopsy

We have already described how IVF progressed from being a treatment for tubal damage to being a panacea for virtually all forms of subfertility. In the 1990s, the role of IVF expanded to include prevention of transmissible genetic disease. It was discovered that an early embryo (at the eight-cell stage on about the third day of development) could have one or two cells (blastomeres) removed without upsetting its development (see Figure 6.5).

1. **Stimulation:** FSH hormone is administered to stimulate the ovary to make several follicles, rather than just the one usually produced in a natural cycle. This is COH.
2. **Monitoring:** The follicular development is monitored using ultrasound and sometimes hormone measurements to assess follicular maturation. This is then triggered by administering a hormone with LH-like activity.
3. **Oocyte collection:** About 34–38 hours later, the oocytes are collected through the vagina using ultrasound control (Figure 6.2).
4. **Sperm preparation, insemination and culture (IVF):** The sperm is pre-prepared and is either mixed with the oocytes, or the oocytes are injected with a single sperm (ICSI), after which the embryos are cultured in vitro for several days.
5. **Embryo transfer:** An embryo is chosen and transferred into the uterus (ET). Today, usually only a single embryo is transferred.
6. **Embryo cryopreservation:** If there are embryos remaining that are good enough to freeze (i.e. they look like they will survive freezing and thawing), these can be frozen and stored in liquid nitrogen to be used in the future.

Table 6.2 The six steps of an IVF cycle

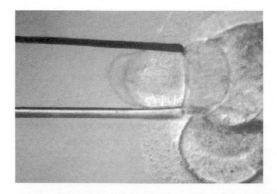

Figure 6.5 The removal of a single blastomere (cell) from an eight-cell embryo.

These cells could then be analysed; initially for complete chromosomes to diagnose if the embryo had an abnormal number of chromosomes (aneuploidy). Each cell of an embryo contains 23 pairs of chromosomes: numbered 1–22, with either two X chromosomes (females) or an X and Y (males). If there is an extra chromosome (i.e. three) in any of these 22 groups, it is called trisomy. The most common is called trisomy 21, in which three number-21 chromosomes are present, and this condition is known as Down's syndrome. Initially only a few chromosomes could be identified using fluorescent in situ hybridisation (FISH), and testing was performed for those that most commonly were abnormal. This technique was first used for medical gender selection using FISH for the X and Y chromosomes.

This enabled identifying male and female embryos from couples who carried serious X-linked diseases (where the 'bad' gene is on the X chromosome) like muscular dystrophy and haemophilia. This enabled transferring only female embryos that would have two X chromosomes, so that the healthy X would compensate for the one carrying the diseased gene. While this prevented passing on the condition, it was not ideal because 50% of the embryos discarded because they were male would have been completely healthy. Furthermore, 50% of the female embryos selected for transfer would carry the condition and the gene would keep propagating in the community. Nevertheless, this was the first successful application of preimplantation genetic diagnosis (PGD) in humans. This was followed by multi-probe FISH protocol (using different coloured markers for each chromosome tested) that enabled simultaneous analysis of several chromosomes in the one cell.

Apart from trying to identify embryos that carried sex linked diseases, the technique of preimplantation genetic screening (PGS); that is, testing blastomeres to make sure the embryo had a normal complement of chromosomes (euploidy) was introduced. This enabled identifying trisomy (three rather than two) or monosomy (only one rather than the normal pair being present) of chromosomes that were known to cause miscarriage, or result in late term fetal mortality, or disability at birth.

The next important change that was developed in about 2010 was biopsying the embryo five days after insemination when it contains about 100 cells (blastocyst biopsy). Blastocyst biopsy had the advantage of providing more cellular material for analysis. Consequently, blastocyst biopsy has been increasingly favoured in recent years. The disadvantage of blastocyst biopsy is that the embryo must be frozen, the result of analysis obtained and then the warmed blastocyst replaced in a subsequent cycle.

The whole concept of PGD was initially proposed to identify embryos affected with serious genetic diseases for couples who carried heritable mutations caused by a single 'bad' gene. The technique of single-cell DNA amplification by polymerase chain reaction (PCR) became the basis of identifying these 'bad' genes, and embryos containing them would not be transferred. Couples who carry these genes can now produce embryos by IVF, the embryos can be tested by PGD and only those that do not contain the suspect gene transferred, enabling the prevention of many inherited diseases.

Today, testing embryos for chromosomal normality (euploid) is called PGT-A and testing for abnormal single genes PGT-M. PGT-A will be considered further in the section, 'Add-ons to Improve Outcome.

Add-Ons to Improve Outcome

The birth of Louise Brown required over 100 ETs, giving a success rate of under 1%. The first series of IVF babies born using stimulated cycles (nine in total) by the author and colleagues' Monash University team in 1981 (the fourth to the twelfth IVF babies in the world) was achieved after 152 oocyte collections and 92 embryo transfers. This gave a success rate of between 6% and 10%. While this showed that IVF could be applied to medical treatment, the efficiency had to improve before it became accepted therapy.

The initial approach was to transfer several embryos, and thus increase the chance of at least one implanting and a baby being born. It then became apparent that this would result in multiple pregnancies with all their associated complications, so consequently the number of embryos transferred has now reduced to usually a single-embryo transfer, with freezing the remainder of embryos that appear able to survive the process of freezing and thawing/warming.

There have been many other strategies used with the hope that they would improve pregnancy and take-home baby rates. Unfortunately, few of these have been proven to be beneficial. It must also be remembered that, for most patients, having a cycle of routine fertility treatment is effective without using any treatment 'add-ons', also known as 'supplementary', 'adjuvants' or 'embryology treatments'.

The current approach to assess the effectiveness (efficacy) of medical treatments is to use evidence-based medicine (EBM). The principle of EBM is that a well-constructed clinical trial should show that the new treatment is better (or at least as good as, if it has other benefits such as cost or fewer side effects) than the existing treatment. This requires what is called a randomised controlled trial (RCT). What we mean by RCT is that susceptible patients are randomised into those who have the old treatment, and they are compared to the group that are randomly selected to have the new treatment.

Enough patients must be followed up in both groups that a statistically significant difference can be detected. Unfortunately, these studies are difficult to perform and few of the add-ons have been shown to significantly bring improvement to pregnancy rates. Many of them are expensive or uncomfortable, so caution is indicated when considering these add-ons. It might be more effective to pay for multiple routine treatment cycles, rather than spending large sums of money on treatment with add-ons that haven't been proven to be effective.

The Human Fertilisation and Embryology Authority (HFEA) in the UK have tried to simplify the understanding of these treatments by using a traffic-light system: green for those that have been shown to be effective, amber for those where effectiveness is undecided and red if it has been shown that the treatment is ineffective. However, if we consider the common add-ons listed on the HFEA system, there are no green traffic lights. In contrast, there are several red lights on techniques where there is no evidence that they improve the chance of having a baby, but which are used in IVF clinics every day.

The following 'add-ons are all classified as red in the HFEA traffic light system; that is, that there is evidence that the treatment is ineffective.

Assisted Hatching

The assisted hatching (AH) technique became popular in the 1980s, and the principle was that drilling a hole in the outside covering layer (ZP) of the oocyte was thought to facilitate the release of the embryo and subsequent implantation, irrespective of the underlying cause; be it thickening/hardening of the ZP or lack of resilience.

Unfortunately, several RCTs have shown that it was not effective. It is possible it may help some couples in special groups (e.g. older women), but this cannot be supported by any evidence.

Immunological Tests and Treatment

The immunology of implantation of an embryo is a very complicated process. It was hoped that altering the immune system may improve implantation and pregnancy rates. Several types of immunological tests have been postulated to be helpful in diagnosing an 'immunological problem', but none of these tests have been shown to correlate with outcome in controlled trials. Consequently, there is no evidence from controlled trials for any immunological treatment (in healthy women) that have shown an improvement. This includes the use of steroids (prednisolone, dexamethasone, and so on), intralipid, intravenous immunoglobulin, TNP-α blocking agents (e.g. infliximab, adalimumab, etanercept). The exception is that immunosuppression should be continued for women with immunological disorders, and they need to continue these for their general well-being.

Intracytoplasmic Morphologically Selected Sperm Injection

While standard IVF still allows the oocyte to select the sperm that fertilises it, with ICSI it is the embryologist who chooses the sperm. It has been suggested that, by inspecting sperm with a very high-powered microscope with 6000-fold magnification (intracytoplasmic morphologically selected sperm injection; IMSI), 'superior' sperm could be selected. However, the outer appearance of a sperm does not reflect normality. Not surprisingly, RCTs have not shown a better outcome using IMSI. Again, there may be some subgroups for whom the technique may be effective, but these have not been identified.

Physiological Intracytoplasmic Sperm Injection

Physiological intracytoplasmic sperm injection (PICSI) is another technique that hopes to identify the best spermatozoa to use in ICSI. The process involves using hyaluronic acid to which the 'better' sperm bind and can then be selected for ICSI. Unfortunately, evidence from a large RCT showed no significant improvement in outcomes using PICSI.

Intrauterine Culture

The culture of the early embryo takes place in culture medium in the laboratory in an incubator. With intrauterine culture, the early embryo is cultured in a special device, which is inserted into the uterine cavity for several hours. There is no evidence that intrauterine culture improves the chance of pregnancy. Furthermore, even in natural conception, this early development takes place in the Fallopian tube and not in the uterine cavity.

Preimplantation Genetic Testing for Normal Chromosome Content

There is no doubt that, if an embryo has an abnormal chromosome make up – too many or too few (aneuploidy) – it will not be able to form a normal pregnancy. It therefore was predicted that carrying out PGT-A and not transferring aneuploid embryos should result in a better pregnancy/birth rate. Unfortunately, there is no evidence from RCTs that this is the case. There are several reasons for this. First, the number of euploid embryos formed within a batch of embryos will not be increased by PGT-A, and the abnormal ones declare themselves by not forming a viable pregnancy. Second, the number of embryos available for transfer will be fewer. Third, some normal embryos may not be successfully analysed. Fourth, some normal embryos may be damaged by the process. Consequently, PGT-A for euploidy is not recommended for the average patient. There may be some groups (e.g. the older patient, or patients with previous pregnancy losses, previous pregnancy with aneuploidy or multiple unsuccessful transfers) for whom PGT-A is recommended. We must not confuse PGT-A and PGS for inheritable diseases, which of course is definitely indicated for appropriate couples.

The following add-ons have been given an amber rating by the HFEA; in which there is no conclusive evidence as the results of trials are conflicting. This suggests further research is needed, and the add-on should not be in routine use.

Endometrial Scratching

The theory behind this intervention is that scraping or scratching the uterine lining (endometrium) by releasing chemicals or activating genes may stimulate the lining to be more receptive to the transferred embryo in a future cycle.

Initial studies showed conflicting results, but recent RCTs have suggested that there may be a small improvement.

Adding Embryo Glue to the Culture Medium

The addition of embryo glue (hyaluronate) to the culture medium prior to ET was suggested to improve implantation and take-home baby rates, at least by one RCT. The very emotive name of 'embryo glue' was given to this process, which suggests that it sticks the embryos onto the endometrium, which of course is not the case. Supporting studies were of moderate quality and further evidence is needed before this can be considered 'green'.

Freezing All Suitable Embryos, Avoiding Fresh Embryo Transfers ('Freeze-Only' Cycles)"

Freezing all suitable embryos and avoiding fresh embryo transfers is some-times called 'freeze-all' cycles, but this does not describe the process correctly as not all embryos that are developed can be frozen. Only those that are judged to be able to survive the freezing and warming process are frozen (cryopreserved). What is really meant is that no embryos are transferred fresh, all (suitable) embryos are frozen and none are replaced fresh: freeze-only cycle.

Although millions of IVF babies have been born after fresh ETs, some doctors believe that the hormones used for stimulation resulting in high levels of oestrogens may make the endometrium less receptive and consequently decrease the chance implantation. To overcome any negative effect of the stimulated cycle, all embryos are grown to day-five blastocyst stage, and any suitable for freezing are frozen. These embryos are then replaced in a subse-quent cycle, either in a natural cycle, or with an artificial cycle using HRT, as described earlier in the chapter. This would avoid the high levels of oestrogen circulating in a stimulated cycle and may have better implantation and pregnancy rates.

There is some research to support the idea that the chances of having a baby are increased by using frozen ETs (FETs) rather than fresh transfers. It has also been found that the risk of OHSS is lower and there is less chance of a baby conceived in a non-stimulated cycle having low birth weight. The downside of freeze-only cycles is that, after completing a stimulated cycle, no embryos are transferred and there is no chance of conceiving at that time. Also, the subsequent ET must be delayed at least one month, and then involves additional expense. It is also possible that embryos that may have resulted in a live birth if transferred are discarded as not suitable for freezing. Finally, some embryos may be lost if damaged during freezing or warming.

Time-Lapse Imaging While in Culture

With traditional IVF, the embryos are removed from the incubator for a few minutes each day and inspected under the microscope by an embryologist, who assesses and records the development of each embryo, and the number of cells present and their appearance. With time-lapse imaging, the embryos are not removed from the incubator, and instead the system takes thousands of photographs during the embryo development, enabling the selection of the 'best' embryo based on continuous observation rather than just a daily look. Artificial intelligence can also be used by feeding the images into a computer. While this sounds advantageous, RCTs comparing the outcome using time lapse to traditional embryo selection have provided conflicting results. Thus, it is not yet clear whether time-lapse imaging is cost effective, which is why it is still amber on the traffic-light system.

Sperm DNA Damage Tests

Sperm take two to three months to mature. During that time, DNA is susceptible to factors that may cause the strands of chromosomes to break or fragment. It is postulated that sperm with less damage are more likely to result in normal fertilisation. However, the evidence is conflicting, and the results of a sperm DNA damage test are unlikely to affect the outcome of treatment. There are a number of other interventions that have been enthusiastically suggested as add-ons to improve success rates, which are not traffic-light classified by the HFEA. These include the use of dehydroepiandrosterone (DHEA) to improve ovarian function in women who have diminished ovarian reserve. Dr Gleicher from New York has reported an improvement in oocyte yields, and diminished spontaneous pregnancy loss after pre-treatment with DHEA supplementation. Unfortunately, there is little supporting data from other workers to confirm its efficacy.

Growth hormone (GH) has also been suggested as a possible treatment for poor-responding patients as an adjunct during their stimulation with FSH. Although early reports were promising, more recent studies have provided no clear evidence for the role of GH, and most expert bodies do not recommend its use.

Anticoagulants including heparin, low-molecular-weight heparin (LMWH) and aspirin have all been suggested as possible beneficial adjuncts to aid implantation. These medications have been used for the management of early pregnancy loss, and it was postulated that they may improve endometrial receptivity, resulting in higher implantation rates. However, a recommendation from the American Society for Reproductive Medicine is that there is insufficient evidence to recommend them for clinical use.

A very popular add-on is acupuncture, and, although the scientific rationale for the effectiveness is lacking, it has been postulated that it enhances receptivity of the endometrium by enhancing blood flow and quiescence of the musculature. Although several controlled studies of varying quality have been reported, their findings are contradictory. The consensus of expert reviews of acupuncture as an adjunct to IVF cannot be recommended.

The other adjunct that many couples use before and during IVF is traditional Chinese medicine (TCM). Studies have found that 30%–60% of couples having IVF treatment are using TCM, including acupuncture, herbs, massage, dietary changes, tai chi and qigong. They can be provided by several sources such as naturopaths, acupuncturists, pharmacies or from supermarkets. While some have clinical data, these are mostly studies in China published in Chinese and not easily accessible to western readers. There is a lack of robust and standardised clinical data, and again they cannot be recommended.

In Vitro Maturation

Although Louise Brown was conceived in a natural cycle with a single-embryo transfer, it was the adaptation of stimulated cycles that allowed IVF to become an accepted therapeutic treatment. Nevertheless, stimulation can have side effects, and the possibility of treatment without stimulation does appeal to some couples. The technique that has been developed is the collection of immature oocytes from the ovaries of women who have no (or minimal) stimulation, and then culturing them to maturity in the laboratory. The benefits of this regimen include oocytes being collected earlier in the cycle (an advantage if chemotherapy is to follow), avoiding the cost of hormones, no risk of OHSS and avoiding high blood levels of oestrogen (contraindicated in women with oestrogen-sensitive cancers or clotting tendency).

However, although several-thousand children have been born around the world by this technique since the first birth in 1994, it is still considered as experimental by many. The preferred protocol involves a small priming dose of FSH (150 IU for a few days) and aspirating oocytes when follicles are close to but smaller than 12 mm. Some experts give a trigger injection of HCG, but this is not essential. The collection of oocytes is similar to routine IVF, and the yield is usually 50% of follicles aspirated. The oocytes are then matured in special culture media in an incubator. Once mature, the oocytes are injected by ICSI, and the resultant embryos cultured to blastocyst when they are frozen. Embryo transfer is subsequently performed in a HRT frozen-embryo transfer cycle. In the hands of enthusiast units (of which there are few), success rates are claimed to be similar to a standard IVF cycle.

Success Rates

The final question asked is usually: 'What are our chances of success for our IVF treatment cycle?' This does not have an easy answer as there are many factors influencing success. The most important factor is the age of the woman providing the oocytes, but there are many other variables such as the cause for the subfertility, the duration of the subfertility and any complicating factors. Across the board, expected pregnancy rates are 40% per ET for women under 35 years of age, 30% for 35–39 years, about 25% at 40 declining to less than 5% at 44 years of age. In the case of egg donation, the chance of pregnancy depends on the age of the oocyte donor.

The Fertility Society of Australia and New Zealand (FSANZ) has developed an 'IVF Success Estimator' (www.yourivfsuccess.com.au/estimate) using the main factors that are known to be associated with the success of IVF treat-ment, such as the male and female's age, whether they have achieved a pregnancy in the past, the diagnosis and whether they have had previous IVF. The user enters information, which is compared to a large number of couples who have had IVF treatment in Australia with similar characteristics. This gives an estimate (but we must remember there are other factors that influence IVF success) of the chance of having a baby after the first completed stimulated egg collection, meaning the transfer of all embryos (fresh and frozen) from the one oocyte collection.

This data is presented as 'birth' per stimulated cycle commenced. However, clinics may present their data using different parameters. The highest success rate will be reported if positive pregnancy tests per ET are calculated. Data are also sometimes presented per egg collection, but the truest picture is if the pregnancy rate per stimulated cycle is considered. Similarly, the definition of pregnancy is variable. The most relevant statistics are the cycles that result in a baby, referred to as take-home baby rate. Clinics sometime use the positive pregnancy test to give the highest success rate, others when the ultrasound shows a heartbeat at six to seven weeks (viable pregnancy). Assisted reproduction programmes do not report success consistently and rates vary with the definition used. Success must reflect delivery of healthy babies against the burden of treatment cycles undertaken by couples.

The ultimate concept suggested in 2004 to reflect the delivery of healthy babies, was birth emphasising a successful singleton at term (BESST), where only singleton babies, born full term (37–41 weeks) were considered a success.

In summary, care should be taken when looking at statistics. Keep in mind the saying: 'If you torture the statistics for long enough, they will eventually confess.'

The final point in considering success rates is that different clinics may have different patient populations, and they may not be comparing like with like.

7 Fertility Preservation and Other Reproductive Options

Sperm Cryopreservation

The human clinical practice of sperm freezing, storing and thawing was developed using the techniques transferred from animal husbandry. The first human births using sperm frozen were reported in 1954. This soon became accepted practice, and sperm freezing and banking became widely used clinical tools. It was also recognised that the use of chemotherapy and radiotherapy would often cause subsequent male infertility (azoospermia), and that the technology used for sperm banking could be used to preserve the fertility of such men by storing their sperm before treatment. Clinics started to store semen before cancer treatment in the 1970s, and the service is readily available in most cities.

It is also recognised that some men who undergo vasectomy subsequently regret the decision due to changes in circumstances, most often because of meeting a new partner. It therefore seems reasonable as an insurance policy that men should freeze-store some semen prior to the vasectomy. However, this has not become popular, despite its probable cost effectiveness, perhaps because of the difficulty in wanting to store sperm before a vasectomy in case he changes his mind and wants more children (perhaps with a younger partner). Today, sperm freezing is often undertaken in conjunction with IVF as it eliminates the need for the male partner to be present during the IVF treatment. Sperm freezing is also undertaken when small numbers of sperm are obtained by needle biopsy, or open testicular biopsy in men with azoospermia. The frozen sperm can then be thawed and used for microinjection/ICSI when the female partner's oocytes have been collected.

Oocyte Freezing

While embryo freezing was developed to avoid the transfers of multiple embryos, the need for oocyte freezing was driven by the need to preserve fertility for women undergoing cancer treatment. While those with a partner could utilise embryo freezing, to maintain reproductive autonomy, oocytes had to be frozen on their own. An oocyte is a much bigger cell than a sperm and, consequently, it is more susceptible to damage by the ice crystals that form during freezing and thawing. Initially, the same technique was used as for freezing embryos: slow freezing with propanediol as a cryoprotectant and storage in liquid nitrogen. A lot of the developmental work was performed in Italy, where embryo freezing was prohibited, but egg freezing was permitted. There were some methodological improvements, but the success rates with the technique were disappointing. The freezing of oocytes was revolutionised by the application of vitrification (described in Chapter 6), and this usually results in oocyte survival of over 90%. Consequently, oocyte freezing has become standard practice for fertility preservation, not only for medical fertility preservation but also what is referred to as social freezing.

Medical fertility preservation was introduced as an option for women who were at risk of losing their fertility due to medical treatment, particularly chemotherapy (treatment for cancer or immunological diseases) or deep X-ray therapy. Such women would go through the IVF process steps one to three: stimulation, monitoring and oocyte collection, but rather than inseminating the oocytes, they are frozen and stored to be used in future. This enabled women to preserve their fertility on their own, and to choose their potential partner any time in the future.

Fertility preservation has also been made available for women who wish to defer having children (social fertility preservation) to a later time when their fertility would be declining. Female fertility decreases once a woman reaches her mid-thirties, but those women who do not have a suitable partner at that stage can now consider freezing their oocytes for future use when they meet a partner. Not only does the chance of conceiving decrease after the mid-thirties, but the chance of conceiving a pregnancy with a chromosomal abnormality (especially trisomy 21: Down's syndrome) increases. If a stored frozen–thawed oocyte is used, the risk of chromosomal abnormality is that of a woman at the age when the oocyte was frozen would have experienced. Therefore, not only is the chance of pregnancy improved, but the incidence of chromosomal abnormality in the offspring is decreased.

While social egg freezing is certainly an option, there is no guarantee that it will even work, let alone that it will provide a family. The best guide to predict the chance of success comes from Oktay's egg-freezing calculator. This is available on the internet, and it enables a woman who is planning to freeze some eggs to predict her chance of having a child with eggs that survive freezing and thawing.

The variables that need to be entered are the woman's age when the eggs were frozen and the number that have survived to calculate the chance of having one baby. For example, a woman who froze eggs at 30 years of age, with eight surviving thawing, would have a 25% – or one in four – chance of having a live birth according to the calculator. If we consider a woman who froze eggs at 35 years of age, with four oocytes surviving thawing, according to the egg-freezing calculator, would have a 17% chance of one live birth using her stored eggs.

Thus, although oocyte freezing does give a chance of having a deferred pregnancy, there is no guarantee. If someone wishes to have two children, and maybe has one early pregnancy loss, a large number of oocytes would need to be frozen to complete her family. To collect and freeze such a large number of oocytes is not feasible.

The other unknown is the proportion of the women who undertake oocyte freezing for social reasons. We do not know how many will actually want to use their preserved oocytes: many may conceive naturally, and others may never meet a suitable partner. Consequently, freeze-storing some oocytes for social reasons is an insurance policy, but, as there is no guarantee of success, like many insurance policies, it may not pay out.

Egg Banking

Egg donation will be discussed later in the chapter, but the ability to freeze oocytes and create an egg bank, similar to a sperm bank, makes egg donation far more accessible.

Embryo Freezing

Since the development of freezing embryos in 1983, the possibility of pre-
serving fertility by creating embryos by IVF, freezing them and then transferring them later became possible. The technique was developed – mimicking
the technology used for animal embryos – in the 1970s by David
Whittingham in the UK, using dimethyl sulfoxide (DMSO) as cryoprotectant,
with slow freezing and rapid thawing. There was a need for the ability to
preserve embryos, as by using COH, several embryos were usually available,
and transferring more than one embryo resulted in multiple pregnancies.
Restricting the number of embryos that were transferred could be better
justified when the remainder could be frozen rather than being discarded.
Very quickly, embryo freezing became widely available around the world,
with acceptable survival and pregnancy rates after thawing and transfer.
Consequently, women who were undergoing treatment that could affect their
fertility and who had partners were able to have this treatment, and many
couples did undertake IVF. This was obviously not an option for women who
did not have a life partner, and the need for oocyte freezing without commit-
ting their oocytes to fertilisation by a male was very real. Fortunately, today,
collecting, freezing and storing oocytes is a realistic option.

Ovarian Tissue Freezing

The technique of freezing strips of ovarian tissue in liquid nitrogen, and then
reimplanting these into rodents with subsequent restoration of ovarian function has been known since the 1950s. These techniques were then applied to
human ovarian tissue, and the first human birth using this technique was
reported in 2004 in Belgium. Since then, hundreds of babies have been born
with this technique. There are two approaches. The most common one is to
implant the thawed ovarian strips into the residual ovary. The second alternative approach is to transplant the tissue into another, more superficial area,
such as the abdominal wall or the forearm, making it easier to recover oocytes
if IVF is required. Ovarian tissue freezing is still considered as experimental by
some experts, although there are a growing number of babies born from this
technique around the world.

The advantages of ovarian tissue transplantation over oocyte freezing are
twofold: first natural conception is possible after the transplant (about half

the babies so far have been born without the need for IVF). Second, natural hormones are restored, although only temporarily, but lasting for many months or some years. Some have advocated the technique to abolish the symptoms of menopausal oestrogen deficiency, as a 'natural' form of menopausal HRT.

One possible danger of ovarian tissue transplantation when it is used for women with cancer is that some of the cancer cells may be present in the strips of ovary that are reimplanted. While this is most unlikely for tumours of the breast or bowel, it is theoretically possible for blood-cell cancers (leukaemia or lymphoma), which can circulate throughout the body. Another downside of fertility preservation through ovarian tissue freezing is that it requires multiple operations. First, the ovarian tissue has to be harvested using laparoscopy, then it has to be reimplanted by either laparoscopy or mini-laparotomy (a small cut in the lower abdomen at the hairline), and then IVF may still be needed to achieve a pregnancy. The advantage is that no hormones need to be administered (especially appropriate for breast cancer), and, as there is no preparation needed, the operation to harvest ovarian strips can be performed within a few hours' notice.

Egg Donation

Egg donation is similar to sperm donation in that a woman who can no longer make oocytes has hers replaced by an oocyte donated by an oocyte donor. Of course, this requires IVF technology, and is quite complicated logistically when fresh oocytes are being used as the two women need to have their cycles synchronised. With the ability to freeze and bank oocytes, egg donation has become much easier. As with sperm donation, the limiting factor is the availability of donors, but for egg donation it is far more invasive as the donor needs to undergo IVF with the associated stimulation, monitoring and surgery. Donors are often known to the recipient and may be a friend or a relative. In many countries, payment to donors for their eggs/sperm is prohibited, with the exception of reimbursement of 'reasonable' expenses. In other countries, for example in the US and some European countries outside the European Union, donors can be paid, and commercial egg donation is possible, and these countries have clinics specialising in 'reproductive tourism'.

The donors are usually young, often university students, and consequently the eggs are fertile and success rates are good. With the ability to freeze and bank eggs, the system is similar to sperm banking. In many countries, including the UK, Australia and EU the identity of the donor is available to the offspring when they reach adulthood, so it cannot be an anonymous donation.

Embryo Donation

As embryo freezing became established and success rates improved, there were couples who completed their families and still had embryos frozen. The option for these families was to have the embryos discarded, donate them for approved research (of which there was very little) or to donate them to another couple. The author and colleagues pioneered the use of embryo donation as early as the late 1990s and found it to be a very worthwhile use of a rare resource. The technique is simple: it is just a matter of undertaking the transfer of a frozen embryo into the recipient woman, either in a natural cycle when ovulation is determined using the LH rise and synchronising transfer, or by using oestrogen HRT to build up the endometrium, adding progesterone, and then transferring on the appropriate secretory day. Unfortunately, we found that less than 10% of couples were prepared to donate their embryos. Their reason was that they did not want somebody else bringing up their children. I can never understand why couples who have experienced the pain of not being able to have children, who have gone through the trauma and effort of IVF, would sooner destroy their frozen embryos rather than giving them the chance of a happy life with, and causing joy for another couple.

Surrogacy

Although reported in biblical times, when Sarah, who was infertile, had arranged for her husband to have sex with her maid, Hagar, and then she raised the child as her own, still surrogacy is the most controversial of the modern methods to have a family. Surrogacy means that a woman carries a baby for another woman who does not have a uterus or is unable to maintain a pregnancy (the commissioning woman).

There are several types of surrogacy, with the options expanding with the use of IVF. Original surrogacy, which requires no or minimal medical involvement, is when a woman who is both the surrogate and the egg donor is inseminated by the male from the commissioning couple at the fertile time of her cycle. She would then be the genetic mother (providing the egg) and the gestational mother who carries the pregnancy and gives birth. The commissioning couple would be the social parents, with the male also being the genetic father as his sperm was used. This type of surrogacy – also known as traditional surrogacy – first achieved worldwide publicity in 1986 with what is known as the Baby M case. Mary Beth Whitehead refused to give up the baby that she was paid US$10 000 to carry, having conceived with her own eggs and Mr Stern's (the commissioning father) sperm. The court ruled that the surrogacy contract was invalid, illegal and perhaps criminal, but ultimately awarded custody to the Sterns as this was thought to be in the best interest of the child. Mary Beth Whitehead was given visitation rights. A similar case in the UK in 1985 was the case of Baby Cotton, where Kim Cotton was inseminated with sperm from the commissioning father and was paid £6500 to carry the pregnancy. The court again awarded custody to the commissioning couple, and the British parliament rushed legislation through to prevent such commercial surrogacies.

Altruistic surrogacy is permitted, with surrogates being paid reasonable reimbursement, which, in practice, can escalate up to £15 000. In the UK, surrogacy contracts remain unenforceable, even in gestational surrogacy (described in the next paragraph), and the surrogate (and her partner if she has one) are the legal parents of the child produced, until parenthood is legally transferred to the commissioning couple.

With the utilisation of IVF, if the commissioning female has functioning ovaries, her oocytes can be collected and inseminated with her partner's sperm. The embryo is cultured in vitro (in the laboratory) and then transferred into the womb of the surrogate, who has either undergone hormone treatment so that her uterine lining is receptive, or, if the embryo was frozen, maybe replaced in her natural cycle at the appropriate time after ovulation corresponding to the age of the embryo. In the latter case, the surrogate is a gestational surrogate – a gestational mother – carrying and giving birth to the baby, but she has no genetic link to the baby. The commissioning couple would be the genetic and social parents. The surrogate 'rents her womb' and has no other connection with the child. American courts have refused custody to surrogates who failed to relinquish the babies they carried on the grounds that the surrogate simply hosted the pregnancy. The situation can be more complicated if oocyte or sperm donors are also involved.

In the UK, surrogacy involves many complicated legal issues. In the UK, the surrogate is the legal mother of the child, unless changed by a parental order from the court. This is not altered even if the eggs and sperm used are from the commissioning couple. Once a court order is obtained, the surrogate will have no further rights or obligations to the child.

It is not possible to know how widespread surrogacy is, but it is estimated that there are more than 1000 cases per year in the US alone, mostly commercial arrangements with a fee of around US$30 000 to the surrogate, with an overall cost to the couple of US$100 000 or more. Cheaper commercial surrogacy is available in some countries such as Thailand, India, Ukraine, Northern Cyprus and where it has not been made illegal. The sociological implications of these new options of forming families have been the subject of a number of studies, and the reader is directed to the book by Susan Golombok (see the reference list at the back of this book). As a generalisation, evidence suggests that the outcomes for these families are no worse than naturally formed families.

Lesbian and Single Mothers

Many women in a female–female relationship wish to have children. There has always been an informal network where males (often homosexual males) would donate fresh semen for lesbian women to self-inseminate (sometimes using a turkey baster) at the fertile time of their cycle. This enabled such women to have children and stay 'below the radar'. The practice of using medicalised inseminations came to the public notice when one woman's story hit the headlines in 1978. A lesbian social support group called Sappho found a doctor who was willing to help with donor insemination of single or lesbian women. When a journalist posing as a lesbian wanting a baby was introduced to this doctor, she wrote a story, which made headline news and brought the issue to the surface.

With the identification of AIDS, the use of unscreened and untested semen became risky, and the need for lesbian and single women to have access to respectable sperm banks became necessary. There was resistance in the UK and Australia to treating single women, and the Medical Procedures Act

1984 in Victoria, Australia specifically limited ART to *married* couples. It took several years for such attitudes to change in these countries, but in the US, semen for self-insemination was available to buy from commercial sperm banks. The semen would arrive in liquid nitrogen with instructions on how to thaw and inseminate.

Today, many countries make mainline fertility services available to single women or lesbian couples. An American psychiatrist, Nanette Gartrell from Harvard Medical School, initiated a study of children born to lesbian couples by using donor sperm. Children were followed up with questionnaires that were used to assess emotional and behaviour problems. They found at that at ages 10 and 17 years old, the children had fewer problems than children in general, and that, at 25 years old, they were psychologically as healthy as their peers. She also reported on sexual identity of these children at 17 years old and found that 5.4% of boys identified as gay, a percentage similar to the general community. None of the girls identified as lesbian. However, by age 25 more of the sons and daughters of lesbian mothers reported some same-sex attraction or experience than their peers, possibly due to a more liberal attitude by their parents.

Gay Fathers

Gay men can become fathers with the help of a surrogate woman. The simplest form is for the surrogate to use her own egg, and then to be inseminated by semen from one of the fathers. This, however, is complicated as parental rights may be disputed. Using IVF technology gives greater security over parental rights (in the US anyway). The children are born by inseminating donor egg(s) with one partner's sperm and then implanting the embryo into the uterus of the gestational surrogate, who has no genetic contribution to the child. Sometimes, the semen from both partners is used to give equal involvement for both fathers. For gay families, the children have two fathers (one of whom is the genetic father), two mothers (a genetic one who was the egg donor and a gestational one who was the surrogate), but no social mother.

A study of 40 gay fathers by Susan Golombok comparing them to 55 lesbian families with children between three and nine years old found that the gay fathers had just as positive a relationship with their children as the lesbian couples, but their children had even lower incidence of emotional problems than the lesbian families' children.

8 Mind over Matter?

Couples who do not have a barrier to conception and have unexplained subfertility sometimes conceive when they stop trying, adopt a child, embark on a new career or go on holiday. It is postulated that in this situation the couple have stopped focusing on achieving pregnancy and, if psychological factors are involved, this may have solved the problem. Psychologists say that women who have a subconscious conflict between motherhood and career may experience this.

Can Anxiety Cause Infertility?

Studies of anxiety levels in couples with fertility problems show higher levels of anxiety. Some studies do show that women who are about to start IVF may be more anxious than control populations. Whether the subfertility causes the anxiety levels to rise, or whether the anxiety causes the subfertility is not easy to determine.

It is believed that anxiety has a negative effect on fertility. In the 1950s, a number of psychodynamic writings considered infertility to be the result of unconscious conflicts in the infertile woman, including the fear of mother-hood and sexuality. Nowadays, most researchers reject the full psychogenic model of infertility. H,owever it is believed that infertility leads to distress, and distress has a negative influence on conceiving. Thus, distress may have a direct effect on IVF outcome through stress-related hormones or immuno-logical mechanisms. Distress may also have an indirect negative effect on outcome through adverse health-related behaviour such as unhealthy eating habits, smoking and alcohol consumption.

During treatment, couples often experience symptoms of anxiety. These symptoms are more pronounced at oocyte pick-up and just before pregnancy testing. Men also show the same pattern of emotional reactions during IVF treatment, but their emotions are usually less intense. Anxiety may act by making the couple unconsciously avoid intercourse during the fertile period, or the woman may develop pain during intercourse as an escape strategy. Anxiety may act through abnormal tubal spasm or by causing unreceptive endometrium. In men, it may manifest as impotence or premature ejaculation, or it may affect sperm quality. These are all hypothetical mechanisms and cannot be explained with current understanding of the physiology of fertility. Anxiety is often caused by conflict, which can be within the relationship or with relatives. There are couples who cannot conceive while living with relatives, but rapidly do so when they move into their own home.

It is important that a couple have the right reason for wanting to start a family. Loneliness, wanting to be loved, proving masculinity or femininity, wanting to hold onto a partner or pleasing parents are all motives that could manifest as covert resistance to becoming pregnant. These problems are hard to admit to oneself, but talking to a third party, a counsellor, a doctor or a close friend may help.

Being Subfertile Is a 'Loss': the Grief Reaction

Not being able to become pregnant, especially once a problem has been identified, represents a 'loss of fertility' and is associated with a grief reaction. There are several stages of a grief reaction with psychological and emotional dimensions, and these are well recognised. See Table 8.1 for the five recognised stages of a grief reaction, as described by Elisabeth Kübler-Ross in 1969.

Denial
Anger
Bargaining
Depression
Acceptance

Table 8.1 The five stages of Grief reaction (Kübler-Ross)

Although they relate to the loss of a loved one, they apply equally to loss of fertility.

The first stage is denial, and with loss of fertility, it is often in the forms: 'They must have made a mistake', 'The test must be wrong'. 'They must have the wrong patient'. It can be hard to believe that an important part of our life is lost. The second stage is that of anger. This is commonly experienced after a loss, and it is part of adjusting to reality with extreme emotional discomfort. Anger is an acceptable emotional outlet for this discomfort. The third stage of the Kübler-Ross model of grief reaction is bargaining. This may include thoughts such as: 'If this problem is cured, I will be a better person', or 'I will never do ... again'. This bargaining is often directed at a 'higher power' such as God. This is the response to the feeling that there is nothing we can do to change the situation and a feeling of helplessness, and a feeling that appealing to something 'bigger than us' may influence the outcome. The fourth stage of denial is depression. This is the stage where the reality of the situation is accepted, as is sadness. Although this is a normal phase of grief, it makes us less sociable, more withdrawn and stops us communicating with others about how we feel, which results in isolation. It is often associated with physical problems such as inability to sleep, loss of appetite and many other symptoms. The final stage is acceptance. This does not mean that the pain has reduced, but it is a stage in which the situation is accepted. While still experiencing sadness, the time has come to move on and explore solutions.

The nature of medical consultations is that the doctor, immediately after making the diagnosis, tends to launch into therapeutic options, and this is at a time when the patient/couple are just starting their grief reaction. Once they have gone through all the stages, they are in a better space to make rational decisions about treatment. At the time of diagnosis, they are probably in shock and find it hard to concentrate. Conversely, the doctor feels that offering possible solutions may make the couple feel better. It is therefore important that the information is repeated, and that written information is provided for later review by the couple.

Another effect of being subfertile is a loss of self-esteem, which can also lead to anger, frustration, depression and self-pity. They may feel embarrassed or inferior to their friends when dealing with them in social situations, and avoid contact, becoming isolated. Often, times like Christmas or 'back-to-school' times are particularly difficult. It is not uncommon to isolate from friends who are pregnant or have young children, and to find it painful to attend family functions with nieces and nephews.

To try and prevent couples racing into complicated treatments, most jurisdictions have introduced statutory counselling prior to IVF treatment. In the UK, the Human Fertilisation and Embryology Act (1990) established that consulting by properly qualified and trained counsellors prior to making an informed consent to ART treatment was compulsory. A similar situation exists in Victoria, Australia.

The Different Types of Counselling

Counselling was defined by the British Infertility Counselling Association in 1991 as: 'A process through which individuals and couples are given an opportunity to explore their thoughts, feelings, and beliefs, in order to come to a greater understanding of their present situation, and to discover ways of living more satisfactorily and effectively. Given this opportunity, they will often change their perspectives, become less stressed and so be in a better position to make informed decisions for the future'.

The treatment of subfertile couples is very much a team approach, and, as along with clinicians (doctors and nurses) and scientists, counsellors are part of the team. Although they have some role in assessment before treatment, their ongoing role is to support couples who have emotional difficulties dealing with their fertility problems and during the difficult process of treatment. Couples are often only partially through the grief reaction when treatment starts, and they can experience anger and frustration during its course. They often feel resentful that something that is a private and personal activity has become quite public. This is often complicated by religious beliefs as several churches, while promoting procreating, are opposed to most forms of ART. There are also ethnic groups who do not approve of such technologies. These can cause feelings of guilt and shame, as well as causing extra conflicts for couples.

Couples are often bewildered by the complexities of choices for treatment and can be apprehensive and frightened by what lies ahead. Medical appointments often feel rushed, and couples may feel inhibited to ask questions from what they perceive as a busy doctor. Counsellors who work in fertility clinics have a good understanding of the technology, and they can help demystify the forthcoming process.

Therefore, fertility counselling has several important areas. First is the statutory role of information counselling. This type of counselling is unusual because it is not initiated by the couple but is a compulsory barrier that has to be overcome before couples can progress. Its aim is to reiterate the technical information provided by the clinician and to ensure that the couple understand what they are signing up for. As anxiety during a clinical consultation may erase some of the information, written information to read at leisure is provided by most clinics. The counsellor can then reiterate the information in what is hopefully a more relaxed atmosphere.

There is also implication counselling where the consequences of treatment for the couple, their offspring and their families are explored. This is particularly important if donor gametes, embryo donation or surrogacy is used (see Chapter 7). It is also important that couples are aware of possible complications of any treatments (e.g. OHSS and surgical complications in IVF), and that, when they sign their consent forms, it is clearly informed consent. Most couples entering an ART programme have only one, maybe two, sessions, lasting 45–60 minutes. It should be in a private, comfortable space.

For couples undergoing fertility treatments, support counselling must be available. The treatment can cause stress and, while all staff at the clinic should be supportive, having a counsellor available to supplement the couple's own strength and resources can help. These sessions should be in a specific location (not in the waiting room or general clinic area), and for reasonable length of time. Additional support can be provided by support groups (see the section, 'Coping with Stress' later in this chapter).

Some couples will need therapeutic counselling if their reactions or symptoms are more profound. This may involve helping them understand the consequences, modifying their behaviour – including accepting the prospects of failure – or reducing stress. Introducing techniques for stress management during treatment is often useful. While it is unlikely that any couple would come to terms with their infertility, counselling can help them cope with their sadness.

Coping with Stress

The first step is for couples to recognise that they are stressed. Professional advice may help, such as counselling for family conflicts, relationship problems or sexual problems. Sometimes the advice of their doctor or a psychiatrist is required. If couples seek professional help, their counsellor will advise stress-management strategies. If couples cope on their own, they may find it useful to read a book on stress management. Often, discussing the issues with a close trusted friend may help.

There are patient-support groups they can join such as Resolve in the US, or Access in Australia, and meeting other couples with similar problems helps them to realise that what they are feeling is not unusual.

Self-help can include partaking in other activities, especially physical activity. Not only is this a diversion, but completing these tasks give a feeling of achievement. Couples should give themselves some 'me' time: reading, going to see a movie, gardening or whatever they find relaxing. Some couples find meditation or yoga helpful.

Will a Holiday Help?

Couples having difficulty conceiving are often told to have a holiday. Although some may succeed in conceiving, studies following up couples have shown that having a holiday does not increase the chance of achieving a pregnancy.

Support Groups

In the early days of IVF, couples felt very much that they were unusual partaking in a 'brave-new-world' experiment. Groups were established very early in the 1980s to provide peer-group support for each other, and to better understand the IVF process by meeting with the clinic staff in information meetings. The Monash IVF support group was known as 'IVF Friends'. Not only did they compare experiences, but they also undertook fund raising, which was very welcome. A national body was later formed in Australia called Access, Australia's National Infertility Network, which became the political authority in debates over funding and approval of new procedures, and it acted as a general representation for patients where it was difficult for individuals to speak out because of confidentiality. In the US, Resolve was formed so that 'people challenged in their family building journey should reach their resolution by being empowered by knowledge, supported by community, united by advocacy, and inspired to act', while in the UK, the Fertility Network offers a wide range of resources and support.

Most countries have similar support groups, and about 30 of these formed the International Consumer Support for Infertility (iCSi). The vision for the iCSi patient leader network is to empower patients to become full partners in ART healthcare and public policy by building effective relationships with providers, governments and media worldwide. Since 1999, iCSi has brought patient leaders together from around the world to better promote access to high-quality and affordable infertility health care. They are working hard in their respective countries to stand up for the rights of patients in accessing infertility treatment.

During IVF Treatment

The first important factor in coping with IVF treatment is to start with realistic expectations. As described in Chapter 6, The FSANZ has developed an 'IVF success estimator' (www.yourivfsuccess.com.au/estimate), using the main factors that are known to be associated with the success of IVF treatment. A prospective couple are advised to visit the website and estimate their own chances before starting so that they have realistic expectations. It is again worth noting, that in real life couples do not expect to conceive the first time they try but embark on a few months of 'trying for a baby'. Some years ago, the author and colleagues constructed a 'life table' to show what expectations couples should have with repeated treatments (see Figure 8.1). The graph shows that the cumulative chance of success increases with each attempt. It also shows the marked improvement in outcomes between 2001 and 2005 and 2006 and 2010.The author and colleagues believe success rates have improved since 2010 when the report was written, and that the figures would be even more optimistic if the report was reconstructed today. As such, the advice is: 'If at first you don't succeed, try, try again' if that is physically, emotionally and financially possible.

Becoming a fertility patient also means that the couple are instructed to undergo a number of tests and procedures, and they may feel they are out of control. To minimise this effect, it is important that the tests and treatments

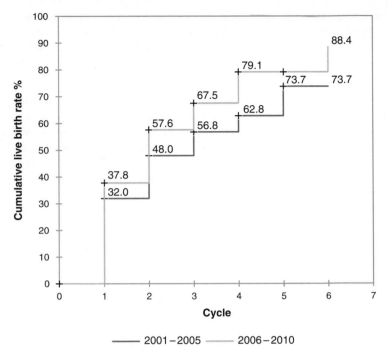

Figure 8.1 Cumulative live birth rates by Kaplan-Meier analysis comparing live birth outcomes for women starting IVF in 2001–2005 with women starting IVF in 2006–2010. Log-rank analysis: p value = 0.006.

and why they are being performed are fully understood. This can be helped by reading all the written material supplied, and asking questions of the medical team about anything that the couple does not understand. The treatment cycle is also quite time-consuming. Appointments must be attended (at times that are often not selected by the couple), blood tests and ultrasound examinations have to be performed with the timing determined by the woman's response, and of course time has to be taken for the oocyte collection procedure and ET. These may also require absences from work. These all have an effect on the couple's social and professional lives. Social activities are often put on hold during a treatment cycle as many couples are not able or willing to share their experiences with others. These commitments also put pressure on the marital relationship, and converting something that used be very private – their sexual relationship – to something that they have to share with others may make matters worse. Partners may disagree about whether to continue treatment or not.

Coping with Unsuccesful Cycles

Even in the best circumstances, fewer than half of couples will be successful with their first attempt. In Chapter 6, it was explained that the IVF process is a like a marathon, with disappointment possible at each step. The woman may not respond to the hormonal stimulation, the timing for egg collection may be inaccurate, not enough eggs may be collected, the male partner may have difficulty producing a semen specimen, insufficient number of eggs may fertilise, the embryos may not develop, the ET may be difficult, and finally the pregnancy test may be negative (more often than not).

Although most couples adjust well to unsuccessful IVF treatment, up to 25% of women report clinically relevant levels of depression after a failed IVF cycle. These feelings usually disappear when a pregnancy is achieved, suggesting that it is just a normal reaction to the treatment. Although some studies have found a positive association between distress and IVF outcomes, the relationship between distress and IVF success rates seems more complex than commonly believed. The popular belief that distress adversely affects IVF outcome may cause feelings of shame and guilt in IVF patients who do not conceive, so clinicians should reassure couples that distress before and during IVF treatment has no significant influence on live birth rates.

Can Counselling Help?

Current understanding is that psychological problems are considered an effect of infertility rather than a cause. Ever since fertility clinics have been established, the provision of psychosocial counselling to couples has been part of the multidisciplinary approach. The role of counselling is to help people understand and cope with issues related to fertility problems and its treatment. A counsellor helps couples to collect and understand all the information that is needed and help with decisions needed for treatment, as well as the emotional and social implications of these decisions,

If IVF treatment is causing emotional distress, counsellors offer emotional support to help couples cope more effectively. Although many couples embarking on IVF may welcome some form of psychosocial counselling, there is a shortage of evidence that psychosocial interventions actually help. Despite the lack of evidence in some clinics and some countries, obligatory pretreatment counselling is obligatory. There is no doubt about the educational value of the counselling sessions that focus on information giving, which include emotional expression and support. These educational interventions are often carried out in a group format, which many couples find reassuring, meeting other couples with similar problems.

Living Without Children: Being 'Child Free'

In a medical consultation, if a fertility problem is diagnosed, it is inevitable that the next step is to explain the available treatment options. Today, with the various types of ART such as IVF, gamete and embryo donors and surrogacy (see Chapter 7) virtually any couple can conceive if they try for long enough. It is therefore easy to get on the cascade of medical consultations, investigations and treatments. Often, professionals who deal with couples are too enthusiastic to solve the problems. However, couples need to ask themselves if that is what they really want. There are social pressures on couples to have children, but a lifestyle that is not centred around children can be happy and fulfilling. Child-free couples are often envied by friends with young children for their independence, freedom and often a more indulgent lifestyle. Focusing on careers, travel and being involved with sports and hobbies are all viable options.

Alternatively, couples may be satisfied by being part-time 'parents' for nieces and nephews, or other children without the need or responsibility of full-time parenting. However, couples should know that, if they wish to pursue having a child, there is every chance they can succeed, one way or another.

Concluding Remarks

The couple who has read this book should now be better informed about how pregnancy occurs and have a better understanding of the various aspects of ART. They also should understand that, in the twenty-first century, there are many ways of parenting and several possibilities for kinship. We have got used to couples divorcing and re-coupling, and of having stepparents and stepchildren.

There are also same-sex couples who are parents, perhaps helped by sperm donation or egg donation and surrogacy. We therefore must be flexible in our understanding of what kinship is. Today, parents can be genetic parents (those whose sperm and egg has formed the embryo that results in a child), birth parents (the woman who gives birth to the child and her partner at the time) or social parents (who bring up and support the child into adulthood).

The benefit of all these options is that virtually anyone can parent by using one or more methods of ART, if they try long or often enough. The saying: 'If at first you do not succeed, try, try and try again' is never truer than for attempts at ART.

It needs to be said again that, when a couple attempt a natural pregnancy, it does not consist of just one attempt, but it involves the discontinuation of contraceptive methods, and it may take several months of unprotected intercourse.

One of the author's couples attempted IVF 37 times before achieving a successful pregnancy. These included six stimulated cycles, after which insurance coverage was only available for minimal stimulation cycles using clomiphene citrate (25 cycles) and natural cycles (three attempts), which resulted in very few oocytes being collected, and these were all disappointing. Fortunately, government policy then extended insurance for more than six cycles, and after two more stimulated cycles where she also had one frozen embryo transfer, she conceived. This treatment took place between April 1991 and March 2002. Her son has now finished school and I have kept in touch with the family. Every time I saw them, she would say: 'Look at Connor now! Every one of those 37 cycles was worth it!' Therefore, the message is: 'While there is life, there is hope', and a couple should keep trying for as long as they can: emotionally, financially and physically.

I hope that reading this book may have made the journey for such couples a little easier. For those who have read the book to have a better understanding of reproduction and fertility, I hope I have succeeded.

Summary of Common Misunderstandings

Particular diets may improve the chances of becoming pregnant. Apart from having a healthy diet and avoiding smoking, excess alcohol and recreational drugs, no dietary factors have been shown to affect fertility.

Certain positions for intercourse enhance the chance of conception. What happens during intercourse makes no difference to conception. As long as semen is deposited into the vagina, nothing else matters.

A woman must have an orgasm to conceive. This is not necessary, even though it is recognised that, during orgasm, the uterus undergoes contractions that may help sperm to travel up into the uterus. As long as the right number of fertile sperm are placed in the vagina at the time of ovulation, they will likely find their way to the egg.

Staying in bed, elevating legs, placing a pillow under one's bottom or resting for a certain time after ejaculation into the vagina improves the chances of getting pregnant. Sperm actually enter the cervix within a minute of ejaculation, so none of these factors are helpful.

Semen 'looks' fertile or 'infertile', for example depending on its volume. The truth is that the volume of a man's ejaculate bears no relation to his fertility. Most of the semen is made up of gland secretions and the volume of the actual spermatozoa is small.

The risk of having a child with chromosomal abnormalities is purely dependent on the age of the mother and paternal age is not relevant. While the maternal age is more significant, abnormalities do increase with the age of the father.

It is said, 'What you don't know doesn't bother you', so it is better for children who were conceived using donor gametes not to be told about their origins. Sociologists believe that honesty is important in a family. If a child finds out by accident rather than being told, it is likely to affect the relationship. With today's genetic testing, this is likely, so being honest is the best policy.

Women who have been diagnosed with PCOS can't become pregnant. Women with PCOS can be reassured that, if the primary problem is that of anovulation, it can readily be treated with OI with an excellent success rate. Should there be additional factors, IVF is the 'fall-back' option, again with a good success rate (see Chapter 6). Importantly, having PCOS does not mean sterility.

If a woman does not menstruate, she cannot become pregnant. This is untrue because ovulation precedes menstruation. If ovulation resumes in a woman who has not been ovulating and has not been menstruating, and if she has unprotected intercourse, she may well conceive without having a period. Women who stop oral contraceptives (the pill) sometimes do not get their periods back (known as post-pill amenorrhoea because they have not resumed ovulation). This is probably not caused by the pill, but by an underlying condition (e.g. PCOS or hyperprolactinaemia), which was masked by the hormones in the pill stimulating the endometrium to shed each time the pill was stopped for seven days: the withdrawal bleed. When they stop the pill, the amenorrhoea is uncovered.

A woman cannot get pregnant if her uterus tilts backwards. As long as sperm can enter the cervix, the position of the uterus is irrelevant.

If a woman's Fallopian tubes are open, they must be working. Fallopian tubes are more than just a 'piece of plumbing'. If the lining is damaged, for example, they may not function adequately.

If a woman has endometriosis, she cannot conceive. Many women with endometriosis do still conceive.

If a woman's tubes are blocked, she cannot ever have children. Fortunately, although repairing blocked tubes only has a low success rate, IVF is now available to overcome tubal infertility.

Once there is a positive pregnancy test, a woman is sure to have a baby. Unfortunately, about one in six pregnancies stop developing. If this occurs under 20 weeks of gestation, the word 'miscarriage' is often used, but the term 'early pregnancy loss' might be more appropriate. If the same phenomenon occurs after 20 weeks of gestation it is called a 'stillbirth'.

Cervical secretions must be killing sperm. This has been suggested for 200 years, but there is no evidence to support it. In fact, we believe that cervical secretions function as a reservoir, protecting the sperm from vaginal acidity, rather than as a barrier.

If a woman moves around after sex, the semen will run out. Sperm enter the cervical mucus within a minute of ejaculation and, although some of the fluid may leak out, plenty of sperm will be available for fertilisation.

IVF was developed for the treatment of damaged tubes and is of no use to overcome unexplained subfertility. The success rates for treating unexplained subfertility by IVF are similar to those for tubal disease.

Once an embryo is implanted into a woman's uterus after IVF treatment, she is pregnant. The embryo has to implant and establish its blood supply before pregnancy can be established. This only happens, at best, about 50% of the time. It is only 10–14 days after transfer that a pregnancy test is performed to see if a pregnancy has been established. Even when a pregnancy test is positive, it is not definite that a woman will have a baby. Unfortunately, one in six pregnancies (whether naturally conceived or by IVF) diagnosed at six weeks do not result in the birth of a baby.

IVF is rarely successful. Over the last forty years, success rates for IVF have significantly improved. While the chance of success is dependent on several factors, the most important is the age of the female partner who provides the oocytes.

IVF is a complicated process. While there are several steps in an IVF treatment cycle, with appropriate explanation and support, it can be managed by most couples.

IVF is just a treatment for infertile couples. This was the reason for the development of IVF, but it has now been extended to allow for preimplantation diagnosis of genetic diseases in embryos, thus enabling selection of unaffected ones.

Freezing eggs and sperm significantly decreases their fertility potential. Current methods of cryopreservation result in excellent survival of both sperm and eggs.

Ovarian tissue freezing is an experimental procedure. With well over 100 babies born around the world using this technique, it can no longer be considered as experimental and it should be an option offered to women who need medical fertility preservation.

Women who cannot use their own oocytes can easily purchase eggs from younger women. In most countries, payment (beyond reasonable expenses) is illegal. There are a few countries where women can be paid for donating their eggs, and these countries have large donation programmes for fertility tourism.

Surrogacy is illegal in most countries. There are many countries where surrogacy is legal, including the UK. However, it involves a lot of complicated legal issues. In particular, the surrogate is the legal mother of the child unless one gets a parental order from the court.

Children brought up in unusual families like two lesbian or two gay parents have more problems when they become teenagers. Evidence from family studies show that these families function just as well conventional families.

Children conceived by IVF are different. Studies of both child development and family functioning have shown that children conceived by IVF are no different to other children. The families function the same as those with naturally conceived children.

A woman may not be able to become pregnant if she is too anxious about it. Anxiety is unlikely to prevent pregnancy, although we do not fully understand how the mind influences conceiving.

The most successful treatment for couples who cannot conceive is to have a holiday. There is no evidence that having a holiday improves the chance of conceiving. Many causes of subfertility are not able to be treated without medical procedures.

Life without children is not fulfilling. This is not so. Many couples who are not parents live meaningful and enjoyable lives.

Fertility treatment is very stressful. While some couples do find treatment stressful, the process can be helped by various stress-management strategies. Understanding what is going on, what is causing the problem and why various treatments are recommended is important. The author hopes that this book will help with improving this understanding.

Glossary

Acrosome reaction	Change in the sperm head before it can fertilise the egg
Adhesions	Scarring between organs
AH: assisted hatching	A method of placing a hole in zona pellucida
AIH: artificial Insemination with husband (partner)	Inseminating a woman with her partner's sperm using an instrument
Algorithm	A series of choices for treatment
Altruistic surrogacy	Being a surrogate without payment
Amenorrhoea	Absence of menstruation (periods)
AMH: Anti-Müllerian hormone	A hormone level that indicates how many potential eggs are left
Ampulla (of the Fallopian tubes)	The open trumpet-like ends of the Fallopian tubes
Androgens	Hormones with a masculinising effect
Andrology	The study of fertility; an andrologist is a doctor who specialises in male hormones/fertility
Aneuploid embryos	Embryos that do not have 46 chromosomes
Antibodies	Blood proteins produced by the immune system
Anticoagulants	Drugs that prevent clotting
Antisperm antibodies	Antibodies against sperm
Appendix	A part of the bowel, which can get inflamed

ART: assisted reproductive technology	Various techniques to help conceive a pregnancy
Asthenospermia	Decreased number of moving sperm (low motility)
Azoospermia	No sperm in the ejaculate
Bacteria	Microscopic organisms that cause infection
BBT: Basal body temperature	The graph of temperature taken each morning on waking
Birth father	The mother's partner when giving birth
Birth mother	A woman who gives birth
Blastocyst	An embryo consisting of about 100 cells at five days of development
Blood–testis barrier	The separation of sperm from the immune system
Bromocriptine	A drug used to treat hyperprolactinaemia
Cabergoline	A drug used to treat hyperprolactinaemia
Cannula	A small or narrow tube
Capacitation	The activation of the sperm to allow fertilisation
Cautery loop	A wire loop through which an electric current is passed
Cervix	The neck of the uterus (womb)
Chemotherapy	Drugs used to kill cells (usually cancer cells)
Chickenpox/varicella	A viral infection
Chlamydia	A bacterial infection, which is a common cause of STIs
Chromosomes	Structures within the nuclei of cells responsible for genetic makeup
Cilia	Small, hairlike structures, which extend from the surface of cells (e.g. in the Fallopian tubes)
Cleavage of embryo	The division of cells in the early embryo
CMV: Cytomegalovirus	A virus that may cause congenital abnormalities if contracted during pregnancy

COH: Controlled ovarian hyperstimulation	Stimulation with FSH in an IVF cycle
Commercial surrogacy	Surrogacy where a woman is paid to carry a baby for another woman
Commissioning couple	A couple who request another woman to be a surrogate
Corpus luteum	The part of the follicle remaining after ovulation
Culture media	A fluid containing specific chemicals to support embryo development in vitro
Cytoplasm	The major part of a cell, which contains a nucleus
Cytotoxic	A compound that kills cells
Cytotrophoblasts	The inner layer of the blastocyst, which then form the the embryo
D&C: Dilatation and curettage	A gynaecological operation to sample/scrape the uterine lining
Danazol	A drug used to treat endometriosis
Deep X-ray therapy	Use of X rays to kill (cancer) cells
DHEA:Dehydroepiandrosterone	A hormone with a masculinising effect
DI: Donor insemination	Insemination of donor sperm
Diagnostic laparoscopy	A keyhole surgery technique to inspect pelvic contents
Diathermy	Electricity-generated heat
Dizygotic twins	Twins that are formed from two eggs fertilised at the same time
DMSO: Dimethyl sulfoxide	A chemical used to protect embryos during freezing
Down's syndrome	A congenital abnormality when three 21 chromosomes are present: Trisomy 21
Ectopic pregnancy	Pregnancy outside the uterine cavity
EDC: Expected date of confinement	Nine months and seven days from the start of the last menses (if regular periods)
Egg bank	A place to store frozen eggs for recipient use
Egg-freezing calculator (Oktay)	A formula that calculates the chance of having a baby with frozen eggs

Ejaculate	The seminal fluid (sperm) containing sperm and prostate gland and seminal vesicle secretions
Embryo	The fertilized oocyte up to six weeks
Embryologist	A scientist who works in an IVF laboratory
Endometriosis	A condition when uterine lining grows outside the uterine cavity
Endometrium	The lining of the uterine cavity
Enzymes	Biochemical substances that speed up metabolism
Epididymis	Part of the duct system between the testes and the vas deferens
Epithelium	A lining of cells in organs
ET: Embryo transfer	The replacement of an embryo after IVF
Euploid embryos	Embryos with a normal chromosome complement of 44 plus a pair of XX or XY
Fallopian tube	A tube passing from the ovaries to the uterus
Falloposcope	An instrument that is used to visualise the inside of the Fallopian tube
Ferning of mucus	Characteristic appearance of fertile cervical mucus under the microscope
Fertile mucus	Stretchy, clear mucus, which has a fern-like appearance under the microscope
Fertile week	The week when intercourse is likely to result in conception
Fertility pills	Tablets used to stimulate ovulation
fertility preservation	Freezing of gametes (eggs and sperm) for future use
Feto-maternal circulation	The blood flow through the placenta, with fetal and maternal circulations separated
Fetus	The developing baby from six weeks until birth
Fibroids	Fibromuscular growth within the uterus
Fimbriae of the Fallopian tube	The finger-like ends of the Fallopian tube

FISH: Fluorescent in situ hybridisation	A technique for identifying chromosomes under the microscope
Flow chart	A series of choices; also known as an algorithm
Follicle	A cyst in which the developing oocyte grows
FSH: Follicle stimulating hormone	The hormone that stimulates oocyte maturation and sperm production
Galactorrhoea	Milky discharge from the nipples
Genetic father	The male whose sperm are incorporated in the baby
Genetic mother	The woman whose eggs are incorporated in the baby
German measles/rubella	A viral infection, which causes fetal abnormalities
Gestational surrogate	A woman who carries a baby for another woman
GH: Growth hormone	A hormone secreted by pituitary stimulating growth
Glycoprotein	A molecule that comprises protein and carbohydrate
GnRH agonist	A hormone that depletes GnRH release
GnRH antagonist	A hormone that blocks GnRH release
GnRH: Gonadotrophin releasing hormone	A hormone that stimulates FSH and LH
Gonorrhoea	An infection transmitted during sexual activity
Gradient centrifugation	A technique of separating particles by high-speed spinning
Granulosa cells	Cells surrounding the maturing oocyte, which secrete oestrogen
Grief reaction	Five stages of grieving after a loss
HCG: Human chorionic gonadotrophin	A hormone produced by the placenta
Heparin	An anticoagulant
HSG: Hysterosalpingogram	A radiological technique to visualise the Fallopian tubes

Hyaluronate	A chemical added to culture media to aid implantation, also called embryo glue
HyCoSy: Hysterosalpingo contract sonography	An ultrasound technique to visualise the Fallopian tubes
Hyperprolactinaemia	Elevated level of prolactin
Hypospadias	An abnormal opening of the urethra on the underside of the penis
Hypothalamic-pituitary-ovarian axis	The hormonal pathway that controls oocyte maturation/ovulation
Hypothalamus	A gland at the base of the brain, which secretes GnRH
Hysterosalpingogram	a radiological examination of the Fallopian tubes
Hysteroscope	An instrument to inspect the uterine cavity
iCSi: International Consumer Support for Infertility	A group of advocates for supporting couples with fertility problems
ICSI: Intracytoplasmic sperm injection	A technique of injecting sperm into the oocyte
Idiopathic	Cause not recognised
Immature sperm	Sperm that need to mature before becoming fertile
Immotile sperm	Sperm that are not moving
Immunological disorders	A person with an abnormal immune system
Implantation	The early embryo establishing its blood supply
In vitro	In a test tube/laboratory
Incubator	A special oven for growing embryos
Interstitial cells of the testes	The part of the testes that secretes testosterone
IVF insemination	The mixing of the oocyte with sperm
IVF: in vitro fertilisation	Growing embryos in a test tube/test tube baby
Karyotype	The chromosomal makeup of an embryo/person
Klinefelter syndrome (XXY chromosomes)	An abnormality in males with an extra X chromosome

Laparoscope	A telescope used to inspect the abdomen and pelvic cavities
Laparoscopy	The process of using a laparoscope
Laparotomy	Inspecting the abdominal cavity after surgically opening it
Leading follicle	The follicle that is destined to ovulate
Letrozole	A hormone tablet that stimulates ovulation
LH peak	A transient (24-hour) rise in LH hormone, which triggers ovulation
LH: Luteinising hormone	A hormone secreted from the pituitary gland
Libido	Sex drive
LOD: Laparoscopic ovarian drilling	A technique for stimulating women with PCOS to ovulate
Luteal phase	The phase of the menstrual cycle after ovulation
Makler chamber	An instrument used to perform a sperm count
Menopause	The end of reproductive life for a woman
Menstruation	The monthly shedding of the uterine lining if no conception takes place
Metabolite	A substance produced during the breakdown of a product
Methotrexate	A chemotherapeutic drug used in treating cancer and some other conditions
Microdeletion of Y chromosome	Missing segments of the Y chromosome
Microdrops	Very small drops of fluid
Microinjection (in IVF)	Injecting with microscopic control, e.g. sperm into the egg
Microsurgery	Surgery that is carried out while looking down the microscope
Minimally invasive surgery	Using telescopes to look inside the body without having to do a formal incision
Monophasic temperature chart	A basal temperature chart where the temperature oscillates around a baseline

Monozygotic twins	Twins formed by an embryo dividing: identical twins
Morphology	Shape
Motility	Movement
Myometrium	The muscle layer of the uterus
Natural family planning	Estimating the time of ovulation to avoid conception
Negative feedback	The ability of a hormone to turn off another
Oestrogen	The predominant female sex hormone
OHSS: Ovarian hyperstimulation syndrome	The overstimulation of follicles, usually by FSH
OI: Ovulation induction	Stimulating ovulation in women who do not normally ovulate
Oligospermia	Sperm concentration below normal (<14million/ml)
Oocyte	Egg: the female gamete
Operative laparoscopy	Operating by visualising inside the body cavity by a telescope-key hole surgery
Orchidometer	An aid to assess testicular volume by comparing the testes to calibrated ovules (the shape of testes)
Osteoporosis	Thinning of bones
Ovarian reserve	The number of potential oocytes remaining in the ovary
Ovulation	The release of the oocyte
PCOs: Polycystic ovaries	A condition in which there are many follicles around the periphery of the ovaries
PCOS: Polycystic ovary syndrome	PCO appearance associated with symptoms
PCR: Polymerase chain reaction	A technique to analyse genetic material
PCT: Postcoital test	A test that inspects the cervical secretions for sperm after intercourse
PGD: Pre implantation genetic diagnosis	A test of embryos for specific genes
PGS: Preimplantation genetic screening	Identifying embryos with abnormal chromosome numbers (aneuploidy)

PGT-A	Aneuploidy screening of embryos during IVF
PGT-M	The screening of embryos for specific abnormal genes
Pinopodes	Tiny protrusions of the uterine lining
Pipette	A fine glass tube used for aspirating fluids
Pituitary gland	The gland in the brain that regulates ovulation, thyroid function and other hormones
Placenta	The afterbirth, which supplies oxygen to the baby
POI: Premature ovarian insufficiency	When the oocytes run out in a woman under 40 years of age
Polyp forceps	Small forceps used to grasp tissue
Polyspermy	When more than one sperm fertilises an oocyte
Positive feedback	The ability of a hormone to trigger another
Pouch of Douglas	The anatomical space between the uterus and large bowel
Pre-testicular azoospermia	A lack of the hormones needed to stimulate sperm production
Premenstrual symptoms	Symptoms due to hormonal changes of ovulation
Primordial follicles	Early developing follicles
Progesterone	The second-most predominant female hormone
Progestogen	A hormone with progesterone-like activity
Prolactin	A hormone that stimulates lactation
Proliferation (of the endometrium)	The growing and thickening of the uterine lining
Proliferative endometrium	Thickened endometrium due to oestrogen
Pronucleus (plural: pronuclei)	The nucleus of a sperm or an egg during fertilisation
Propanediol	A chemical used to protect embryos during freezing

Prostate gland	A gland at the base of the bladder
Pyosalpinx	Fallopian tube containing pus after an infection
Radiology	Examination using X-Ray
Rh: Rhesus factor (blood)	A blood group factor, which is either positive or negative
Salpingitis	Inflammation of Fallopian tubes
Secretory endometrium	The histological appearance of the endometrium after ovulation
Semen	The fluid ejaculated during an orgasm
Semen analysis	The assessment of the fertility capability of semen
Seminal vesicles	Small glands at the base of the bladder, which provide secretions for the ejaculate
Seminiferous tubules	Part of the duct system of the testes
Sims-Huhner test	A postcoital test to see if moving sperm are present after intercourse
Social father	A man who brings up a child
Social mother	A woman who brings up a child
Sperm bank	A storage facility for frozen semen
Spermatozoa	Mature sperm cells
Spermatozoon	A single sperm cell
Spiral arterioles	Uterine arterioles, which flow to the placenta
Standard IVF	IVF where a subsample of sperm is mixed with an oocyte
Sterilisation	The obstruction of the Fallopian tubes or the vasa to prevent pregnancy
STI: Sexually transmitted infection	An infection transmitted during sexual activity
Submucous fibroid	A fibroid protruding into the uterine cavity
Surrogacy	A woman carries a baby for another woman
Syncytiotrophoblast	The outer layer of the blastocyst, which then forms the placenta

Take-home baby	A live birth (usually after treatment)
Testicular azoospermia	Azoospermia when the testicles are unable to produce sperm
Testis	Male reproductive glands
Testosterone	The leading male hormone
Thawing	Defrosting from a frozen state
THS: Thyroid stimulating hormone	A hormone that stimulates the thyroid gland
Thyroid function test	The assessment of thyroid gland function
Time-lapse photography	Repeated photographs used in following embryo development
Trisomy	Three chromosomes of the same type (1–22) rather than a pair
Tubal abortion	A pregnancy that attempts to implant in the tubes but then aborts
Tubal lumen	The cavity of the Fallopian tubes
Tubules	The small tubes within the testes
Tunica albuginea	Capsule of fibrous tissue covering the tubules within the testes
Ultrasound	A medical imaging technique using radar technology
Urethra	The canal from the bladder to the outside
Uterine cavity	The cavity of the womb
Uterus	Womb
Varicocele	Dilated veins around the testicles
Varicose veins	Dilated veins
Vas deferens (plural: vasa deferentia)	Proper name for the vas: the connecting channel from the testes to the urethra
Vasectomy	The blocking off both vasa to prevent fertility
Viable embryo	An embryo that has the potential to grow into a baby
Vitrification	A technique of rapid freezing use for eggs and embryos
White blood cells	Cells in the blood in response to infection
Window of implantation	The days during which the endometrium is receptive to an embryo

X chromosome	Female chromosome: if two are present, this defines a female
XX	Female chromosome makeup
XY	Male chromosome makeup
Y chromosome	The chromosome that defines a male
ZP: Zona pellucida	A shell around the early embryo
Zygote	An early embryo, lasting from fertilisation until blastocyst stage

References

Chapter 1

Hudhud MA, Trew G. The first interview with a new couple. In: Kovacs G. Ed. *The Subfertility Handbook: A Clinician's Guide*. Cambridge University Press, 1996.

Kovacs GT. Infertility – a flow chart approach. *Aust NZ J Obstet Gynaecol* 1979; 4: 220-4.

McLachlan R, Yazdani A, Kovacs G, Howlett D. Management of the infertile couple. *Aust Fam Physician* 2005; 34: 111-17.

Nisenblat V, Norman R. Pre-pregnancy counselling and treatment. In: Kovacs G. Ed. *The Subfertility Handbook: A Clinician's Guide*. Cambridge University Press, 1996.

Chapter 2

Aitken J, Mortimer D, Kovacs G. Eds. Male and sperm factors that maximise IVF success. Cambridge University Press, 2020.

Fainberg J, Kashanian JA. Recent advances in understanding and managing male infertility. *F1000Res* 2019; 8:F1000 *Faculty Rev* 670.

Hsiao W, Schlegel P. Assessment of the male partner. In: Kovacs G. Ed. *The Subfertility Handbook: A Clinician's Guide*. Cambridge University Press, 1996.

Kovacs G, McLachlan R, deKretser D. The management of male subfertility by in vitro fertilisation techniques. *Aust Fam Physician* 1995; 24: 379– 85.

Kay VS, Barratt CLR. The use of donor insemination. In: Kovacs G. Ed. *The Subfertility Handbook: A Clinician's Guide*. 2nd edn. Cambridge University Press, 2011; 148–57.

Kovacs G, Wise S, Finch S. Functioning of families involving primary school-age children conceived using anonymous donor sperm. *Human Reproduction* 2013; 28: 375–84.

Paul J. *New South Wales Infertility Social Workers Group. How I Began: The Story of Donor Insemination.* Fertility Society of Australia, 1988.

Wise S, Kovacs G. Secrecy, family relationships and the welfare of children born with the assistance of donor sperm – developments in research, law and practice. In: Hayes A, Higgins D. Eds. *Families, Polcies and the Law.* 2014; 81–7.

Chapter 3

Billings E, Westmore A. *The Billings Method.* Anne O'Donovan Publishers, Melbourne, 1980.

FertilityFriend.com. International evidence-based guideline for the assessment and management of polycystic ovary syndrome. Monash University, Melbourne Australia, 2018.

Kovacs G, Smith J. *A Patient's Guide to the Polycystic Ovary.* Hill of Content, 2001.

Von Hofe J, Bates GW. Ovulation induction. *Obstet Gynecol Clin North Am.* 2015; 42(1): 27–37.

Chapter 4

Burney RO, Giudice LC. Pathogenesis and pathophysiology of endometriosis. *Fertil Steril.* 2012; 98(3): 511–9.

Endometriosis: diagnosis and management. NICE guideline [NG73]: 6 September 2017. www.nice.org.uk/guidance/ng73p.

ranzcog.edu.au. The Royal Australian and New Zealand College of Obstetricians and Gynaecologists. Endometriosis clinical practice guideline (Australia).

Steptoe PC. *Laparoscopy in Gynaecology.* Livingstone, Edinburgh, Scotland, 1967.

Chapter 5

Fatum M, Laufer N, Simon A. Investigation of the infertile couple: should diagnostic laparoscopy be performed after normal hysterosalpingography in treating infertility suspected to be of unknown origin? *Hum Reprod.* 2002; 17: 1–3.

Kovacs GT, Newman GB, Henson GL. The post-coital test: What is normal? *Brit Med J*. 1978;1: 803.

Ombelet W. The role of artificial insemination with partner semen in an ART program. In: Kovacs G. (Ed). *The Subfertility Handbook: A Clinician's Guide*. 2nd edn. Cambridge University Press, 2011.

Trounson AO, Leeton JF, Wood C, Webb J and Kovacs GT. The investigation of idiopathic infertility by in vitro fertilization. *Fertil Steril* 1980; 34: 431–8.

Chapter 6

Aitken J, Mortimer D and Kovacs G. *Male and sperm factors to maximise IVF success*. Cambridge University Press, 2020.

Edwards RG, Steptoe PC. *A Matter of Life: the story of a medical breakthrough*. Morrow, New York, NY, USA, 1980.

Kovacs G, Brinsden P, DeCherney A. *In-vitro fertilization: the pioneers' history*. Cambridge University Press, 2018.

Kovacs G, Norman R. *How to improve preconception health to maximise IVF success*. Cambridge University Press, 2018.

Kovacs G, Rutherford A Gardner D K. *How to prepare the egg and the embryo to maximize IVF success*. Cambridge University Press, 2019.

Kovacs G, Salamonsen L. *How to prepare the endometrium to maximise IVF success*. Cambridge University Press, 2019.

Min JK, Breheny SA, MacLachlan V, Healy DL. What is the most relevant standard of success in assisted reproduction? The singleton, term gestation, live birth rate per cycle initiated: the BESST endpoint for assisted reproduction. *Hum Reprod* 2004;19(1): 3–7.

Nagy ZP, Shapiro D, Chang CC. Vitrification of the human embryo: a more efficient and safer in vitro fertilization treatment. *Fertil Steril*. 2020; 113(2): 241–7.

Pfeffer N. *The Stork and the syringe: a political history of reproductive medicine*. Polity Press, Cambridge, UK, 1993.

Steptoe, PC, Edwards, RG. Birth after reimplantation of a human embryo. *Lancet*, 1978; 366.

Wade J, Maclachlan V and Kovacs G. The success rate of IVF has significantly improved over the last decade. *Aust N Z J Obstet Gynaecol* 2015; 55:473–6.

Chapter 7

Anderson RA, Davies MC, Lavery SA. Elective egg freezing for non-medical reasons: Scientific Impact Paper No. 63. *Royal College of Obstetricians and Gynaecologists.BJOG.* 2020; 127(9): e113–21.

Audrins P, Holden C, McLachlan R. Kovacs GT. Semen storage for special purposes at Monash IVF 1977–1997. *Fertil & Steril* 1999; 72: 179–81.

Bunge RG, Keetel WC, Sherman JK. Clinical use of frozen semen. Report of 4 cases. *Fertil Steril* 1954; 5: 520–9.

Donnez J, Dolmans MM, Demylle D, Jadoul P, Pirard C, Squifflet J, et al. Livebirth after orthotopic transplantation of cryopreserved ovarian tissue. *Lancet* 2004; 364: 1405–10.

Golombok S. *Modern families. parents and children in new family forms*. Ambridge University Press 2015.

Golombok S. *We are family*. Scribe publications 2020.

www.fertilitypreservation.org/contents/probability-calc. Oktay's innovation fertility preservation & IVF egg freezing calculator.

Wise S. Kovacs G. Secrecy, family relationships and the welfare of children born with the assistance of donor sperm. Developments in research, law and practice. In: Hayes A, Higgins D. Eds. *Family policy and the law*. Australian Government, 2014, 81–8.

Chapter 8

Burns LH, Covington SN, Burns LH. Psychology of infertility. In: Covington SN, Burns LH. Eds. *Infertility counseling: a comprehensive handbook for clinicians*, 2nd edn. Cambridge University Press, 2006, 1–19.

Clifford J. Counselling In: Serhal P, Overton C. Eds. *Good clinical practice in assisted reproduction*. Cambridge University Press 2004, 266–76.

Malina A, Błaszkiewicz A, Owczarz U. Psychological aspects of infertility and its treatment. *Ginekol Pol* 2016; 87(7): 527–31.

Figure Credits

Index